Natural Choices for
Fibromyalgia

Natural Choices for Fibromyalgia

Discover Your Personal Method for Pain Relief

by:
Jane Oelke, N.D., Ph.D.

Publisher:
Natural Choices, Inc.
Stevensville, Michigan
www.NaturalChoicesForYou.com

Although the authors and publisher have exhaustively researched all sources to ensure the accuracy and completeness of the information contained in this book, we assume no responsibilities for errors, inaccuracies, omissions, or inconsistency herein. Any slights of people or organizations are unintentional. Readers should use their own judgment or consult a holistic medical expert or their personal physician for specific applications to their individual problems.

Printed in the United States of America.
ISBN 0-9715512-0-0

Library of Congress Number 2001097720

Acknowledgements

Thanks to the participants in the bio-chemical research study, the students in the seminars I have taught, and my clients for enlightening me in the many aspects of Fibromyalgia and the opportunities available in natural health to help reduce the symptoms.

I also want to thank Florence Mundt, a client, a friend, and the person who helped me edit this book. Her knowledge of fibromyalgia encouraged my interest in doing the research project, and following up with publishing this book.

Additionally, I want to thank the health practitioners and Service Coordinators at the Holistic Alliance in St. Joseph, Michigan. As a practitioner there myself, I had the ability to perform the research study with the help of their referrals and marketing.

Of course, I want to thank my husband and children, who put up with me while I was dedicating my energy toward completing this project.

Table of Contents

Part I

Part II

Dedication

This book is dedicated to the volunteers who were part of the bio-chemical research study. Those people were willing to try something new to educate themselves about their own health issues.

❧1❧

Part I

What Exactly is Fibromyalgia?

More and more people are being diagnosed with fibromyalgia syndrome everyday. If you are reading this book, you either have fibromyalgia, or you probably know someone who has fibromyalgia, and want to help them know more about it. Too often we are told there is nothing that can be done to relieve the pain of fibromyalgia. The purpose for writing this book is to give people hope. Real differences in how they feel can be made through some relatively simple changes in lifestyle. Since no explanation of any one specific cause of the chronic pain found in fibromyalgia patients exists, we will be looking at various imbalances in the body that often produce pain. Some scientists believe that fibromyalgia may be caused by an injury or trauma. Others believe it is caused by long-term metabolic and nervous system disorders. There are others that believe it is a result of unresolved emotions that become trapped inside the muscle tissue. To effectively assist people who suffer from fibromyalgia syndrome, it is necessary to discover what is really happening in the body.

This book will specifically look at metabolic imbalances and ways to improve the metabolism so that the painful symptoms can be relieved. We will look at how fibromyalgia is diagnosed and what other symptoms are also associated with fibromyalgia. Then we will look at what effects environmental stress has on the metabolism, and how to measure the effects of this stress. We will see that the environment affects many different areas in our lives. The environment we live in influences our health by what we breathe, eat, and drink daily. If our metabolism is not strong enough, these stresses will build up gradually, creating symptoms in various parts of our bodies.

In this book, we will learn how daily nutritional choices either bring in sufficient nutrients for our body to rebuild tissue, or break down tissues due to excess acids in our system. We will discover the source of free radical activity that essentially causes our bodies to "rust", or age more quickly. We will also look at the acid and alkaline balance in our tissues, and learn to tell with simple saliva and urine testing, the direction of our health.

Even though everyone is affected by stress, the health of our metabolism will determine our susceptibility to certain disorders. We will discover common symptoms that relate to metabolism imbalances, and relate them to the known benefits of nutritional supplements and natural health techniques. We will look at nutrition, homeopathy, exercise and bodywork. And you will learn how to recognize which techniques and remedies will benefit you most. All of the information is designed to help people with fibromyalgia; yet, also assists those who want to be healthy and prevent any type of chronic disease.

Throughout these pages the results of a research project will be explained. This research project was conducted in order to discover which types of metabolic imbalances lead to symptoms of fibromyalgia. Looking at the research results and comparing the symptoms of fibromyalgia will enable us to determine which types of natural remedies will be the most valuable and beneficial. Applying this information will make it easier for you to recognize your own needs and develop a program that will most benefit you.

❧2❧

The Philosophy of Natural Healing

Many people turn to natural health techniques to help with fibromyalgia symptoms. Natural health techniques work with the innate intelligence our bodies have to stay healthy. This inborn inner wisdom of the body directs and controls every function of every cell. When we have symptoms, they are warning signals from this innate intelligence that our state of health is being compromised. Symptoms are beneficial indicators that we have caused stress to a certain part of our body, and our innate intelligence is working to correct it. For example, when we have a "cold", the runny nose is a cleansing reaction to a toxic build-up that has occurred. If we suppress these cold symptoms, the body does not have a chance to heal fully, causing a re-occurrence, a deeper imbalance, or disease process later on. Asthma is one of the deeper imbalances of suppressing cold symptoms for a length of time.

In natural healing, a diagnosis is not necessary to discover the treatment protocol. A diagnosis is created from a group of symptoms that are related. By labeling a diagnosis the patient believes that they have a specific disease process. Yet, unless the doctor knows _all_ of the symptoms that are happening, a correct diagnosis is not commonly found. Patients do not get better by knowing the disease name. They may lose hope when a diagnosis is made for a supposedly incurable disease. Practitioners who do natural healing techniques do not diagnosis a disease name. By looking at the specific symptoms of each individual, they recognize imbalances that are occurring and use remedies and/or hands-on techniques to stimulate the innate natural healing ability to bring the body back towards health. This is more than simply prevention of disease; it is actually supporting and maintaining a consistent state of health.

The body's innate intelligence produces symptoms as our warning signal that we are doing something to disturb the natural balance within the body. If the body has the intelligence to produce a disease profile, once the cause is removed, it is also capable of reversing the process and creating health. The body functionally attempts to maintain health and compensate as best it can under the circumstances. To many of us, this compensation causes symptoms that relate to disease profiles. When the disturbance is removed, whether it is physical or emotional, the cells in the body will change their function and return to health. Usually, the longer the body is in the compensation stage, the longer it will take to reverse the symptoms.

Of course, the healing ability depends on the vitality of the body. By definition, the vitality of the body refers to the overall energy level of the body, how well blood circulates nutrients into the cells, and how free the tissues are from toxins. The greater the vitality, the more energy the cells will have to release the toxins and remove them from the body. The skin and mucus membranes will be the most common ways toxins will exit when the vitality is high. When the vitality is lowered, due to an increase in stress or toxic buildup, the body does not have the energy to release toxins and will store them in the tissues causing congestion and pain.

When you are healthy, you are physically, mentally, and emotionally in an optimal state of well-being. Your body is always doing its best to stay in this healthy state. You use your available reserves to keep the metabolism in the best condition possible. Some fibromyalgia patients find this hard to believe. It is difficult for them to believe the pain associated with fibromyalgia is really a warning sign telling them to do something different than what they are doing now.

Research Project Explanation

Throughout this book we will be looking at the results of a biochemical test research project. This project was conducted to effectively measure the relationship of symptoms found in fibromyalgia clients to metabolism imbalances. This research project was performed using 50 volunteers who had been diagnosed with fibromyalgia, and 50 other clients. Test results for other clients, who had not been diagnosed with fibromyalgia, were used as the control group. By comparing the fibromyalgia client's readings, with the control group's readings, we were able to obtain a better determination of the metabolic imbalances that accompany fibromyalgia.

I conducted this research project and wrote this book as a result of the needs of many people that I have interacted with as a naturopathic doctor. As a Doctor of Naturopathy, I focus on helping clients improve their health. While my specialty is homeopathy, I have done biochemical nutritional testing for the last few years. My previous background as a research engineer has provided me with extensive interest in scientifically demonstrating proven ways to help people. The idea for this project came from a seminar I taught to nurses called Natural Choices for Fibromyalgia. Much of the information presented in the seminar correlated metabolic imbalances to fibromyalgia symptoms. When working specifically with clients who were diagnosed with fibromyalgia, most of the relief came when the client was able to improve their metabolism. Therefore, this project was designed to find specific correlations between biochemical test results and fibromyalgia symptoms.

To understand the variety of differences between each person diagnosed with fibromyalgia, every participant in the research project filled out a questionnaire. Information requested in this questionnaire included their age, their date of diagnosis of fibromyalgia, the number of tender points that tested positive, and the locations of pain. The purpose of the questionnaire was to make sure that all of the participants did understand how fibromyalgia was diagnosed and to confirm that they actually have the syndrome. Volunteers who mentioned that their pain was only in one location during the screening process were not part of the study. Fibromyalgia pain has to be located in specific areas of the body as described in the section pertaining to diagnosing fibromyalgia.

Fibromyalgia affects mostly women in their forties and fifties. Of the 50 participants who were part of the fibromyalgia group, 4 were men, and 46 were women. The average age for the participants was 49.7 years old. The ages of the participants ranged between 19 and 85 years old. As people get older they are more prone to fibromyalgia symptoms. You will understand why as we explore the various possible causes of fibromyalgia.

This project tested urine and saliva pH levels, adrenal stress, malabsorption levels, oxidative stress, and vitamin C and calcium levels. Other biochemical nutritional tests that were also completed, but are not included in the results of this study, include a carbohydrate level test, a specific gravity score, and a conductivity score. The results of these other tests were very similar between the fibromyalgia group and the control group. Each explanation of the seven tests that are included in this research study will be explained throughout the rest of the book in the corresponding sections.

❧4❧

How Do I Know If I Have Fibromyalgia?

By definition, Fibromyalgia is a chronic disorder characterized by widespread muscle, ligament, and tendon pain, with stiffness and tenderness on touch, lasting longer than three months, usually accompanied by fatigue, anxiety and/or depression. Fibromyalgia is diagnosed by counting the number of specific tender points that occur in precise, localized areas, particularly in the neck, spine, shoulders, and hips. In January of 1993, the World Health Organization officially declared fibromyalgia syndrome as the most common cause of widespread chronic muscle pain. The World Health Organization stated that people with this syndrome might also experience other symptoms such as headaches, insomnia, cold sensitivity, restless leg syndrome, morning stiffness, irritable bowel syndrome, anxiety, and depression.

Fibromyalgia is called a syndrome, not a disease, since it represents a group of common nonspecific disorders characterized by pain, tenderness, and stiffness in muscles, ligaments, tendons, and adjacent connective tissues. Muscles, ligaments, tendons, and connective tissues are considered "fibrous" tissues. "Myalgia" is a medical term that indicates pain in the muscles, while "myositis" indicates inflammation of the muscle tissues. Fibromyalgia used to be called fibromyositis. However, inflammation is not the cause of fibromyalgia pain. Therefore, the term "fibromyalgia" is used to diagnose pain found in the fibrous tissues, muscles, ligaments, tendons, and connective tissues from non-specific causes. Any of the fibrous tissues in the body may be involved, but the most common sites include widespread pain in the head, neck, shoulders, low back, hips, thighs, and knees.

According to the American College of Rheumatology, fibromyalgia affects 3 to 6 million Americans. The majority are women between the ages of 25 and 50 years old, with females out-numbering males by 6:1.[1] The exact cause of fibromyalgia in this commonly female age group has not been determined. Emotional factors are being looked at, along with physical symptoms.

Many fibromyalgia patients often hold stress inside, and may appear tense, depressed, or anxious. The symptoms are often induced and/or intensified by physical or mental stress, mental overactivity, sleep disorders, physical or emotional trauma, depression, exposure to dampness, heat, or cold, and occasionally by another disease process.[2] A viral or other systemic infection may bring on the syndrome in someone who is susceptible due to a weakened immune system. Patients often trace the onset of symptoms to an acute event or viral-like illness. Fibromyalgia may also be a complication of hypothyroidism or diabetes. Men are more likely to develop localized fibromyalgia in association with a particular occupational or recreational strain, or as a complication of sleep apnea.[3] All of these physical and emotional factors will be looked at in the following chapters.

Pain is the most common symptom of fibromyalgia. Fatigue is the second most common symptom associated with fibromyalgia. This fatigue is both physical and mental. Physically, the muscles feel tired due to low energy reserves. Any normal activity, like shopping, walking up stairs, and routine household responsibilities, can tire the body easily. Mental fatigue includes concentration problems, confused thoughts, and memory weakness. People with fibromyalgia tend to become more forgetful and absentminded than the average person. This happens because the brain is so busy being bombarded by pain signals, it has very little energy left to perform cognitive thinking. Headaches were also common in the participants in the research study. The headaches can feel like tension or migraine headaches. Tension headaches are the result of muscle contractions that usually begin in the neck, and travel up into the head area. Sleep disturbances are also common symptoms. Trouble falling asleep, or frequently waking throughout the night, does not allow the body the precious time required to restore itself. Dry eyes are common visual problems.

Numbness and tingling, especially in the arms and legs, are common neurological disorders associated with fibromyalgia. Tingling may affect the hands and feet with feelings similar to carpal tunnel syndrome, or the sensation as if they were asleep. This can affect the ability to use the hands or walk normally. Dizziness is another neurological disorder associated with fibromyalgia. Light-headedness and balance problems are the cause for lack of coordination. Weakness is another neurological complaint. This loss of strength and stamina creates deeper feelings of fatigue. Leg cramps in the calves, or restlessness in the legs when in bed at night, are also commonly associated symptoms of fibromyalgia.

Eighteen Tender Points

Everyone feels pain at some time in their lives. Pain is a normal response of our nervous system to a danger in our environment. The normal transmission of pain begins at specialized nerve endings in the skin, muscles, bones and other tissues. When heat from a hot stove touches our skin, the specialized nerve endings on our hands respond by releasing neurotransmitters that create tiny electrical currents through the spinal cord and into our brain. We do not realize the sense of pain until it reaches our brain, which happens in just milliseconds. This realization of pain also sends back a signal to our motor nerves in our hands to pull away from the hot stove.

The pain of fibromyalgia is different than this reactive pain response. Even though each person perceives pain differently, and can accommodate certain levels of pain, the pain of fibromyalgia creates a persistent pain that cannot be ignored. It is opposite of the normal accommodation we usually have for pain. For example, when we get into a hot tub, it is very hot at first, then when our body gets used to the heat, it accommodates or adapts to the heat. However, in fibromyalgia, the nervous system is not able to adapt to painful responses. When the pain becomes continuous and it is difficult to find anything to relieve the pain, then it is then time to check the correlation of the persistent symptoms to those of fibromyalgia syndrome.

Fibromyalgia is difficult to diagnose because many of the symptoms mimic those of other disorders. Muscle soreness in one spot, like the neck or lower back, cannot be diagnosed as fibromyalgia. The doctor does have a set of qualifications that differentiates fibromyalgia pain from other types of pain. A diagnosis of fibromyalgia is first based on a history of chronic, widespread pain that persists for more than 3 months. There are different types of pain that are commonly found in fibromyalgia. Some people experience aching pain, others feel sharp, stabbing pain sensations throughout their body. Other people feel burning pain, and some people feel a combination of all these types of pain. The American College of Rheumatology has designed the criteria to diagnosis fibromyalgia for physicians. Patients must fit both criteria to be diagnosed with fibromyalgia.

First, pain has to be spread throughout the body. The pain cannot be located in just one area, such as one shoulder, but needs to be found in all areas of the body, including above and below the waist, and on the right and left sides of the body. This general pain must have existed for at least 3 months.

Secondly, tender, painful spots must be present in at least 11 of the following 18 points when the tissues in these areas are pressed. These points are explained below along with a diagram.

- On the back of the head at the lower edge of the skull, on both sides of the spine.
- Sides of the neck along the crease between the head and neck.
- Mid-point on top of the shoulder in the muscle along the back edge of the shoulder called the trapezius.
- On both sides of the spine, in the middle of the upper back just above the scapula or shoulder bone.
- On the front between the first and second rib in the upper chest area on both sides of the sternum.
- On the inner side of the lower arm, about two inches down from the fold in the elbow.

- Lower back, near the dimpled area of the backside.
- Along the side of the body in the middle hip area.
- Inner side toward the back of the knee.

These points should be pressed lightly and then pushed more strongly with a thumb or tip of one finger with up to two pounds of gentle force. Usually just by lightly touching some of these points you will know if they are painful. These points must not be just tender, but must be painful on touch. Count the number of points, then record where they are located and the degree of pain. This will help you determine when 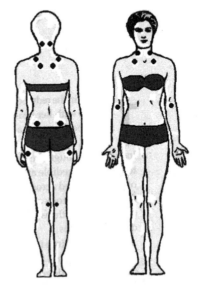 you are feeling better, as the number of points and the intensity of the pain is lowered.

These tender points are painful specific sites in muscles, ligaments, tendons, and other soft tissues of the body. The listed tender points are the most commonly painful areas. There are other areas of the body that are often painful. The other common areas of pain are in the head, and along the legs and arms. In some of these tender places, you will be able to feel nodules or tight bands that feel like a firm lump or "knot". Other painful spots are at insertion points of muscles into tendons and bones. Often the painful sites move around and can be related to muscle spasms.

In the research study, the most common area of pain was in the neck and shoulders area. In fact, 70% of participants indicated pain in the neck area, and 80% of the participants indicate pain in the shoulder area. The second most common area was the lower back where 72% indicated chronic pain. The other areas where research participants indicated the most chronic pain were in the head, as headaches, and in the elbows and knees. These numbers are in direct correlation to the numbers found by the American Academy of Pain Management. They list the frequency of pain in the tender points to be found most commonly in the shoulders (84%), upper back (74%), knees (74%), lower back (62%), elbow area (62%), and neck (56%).

Relationship with other Diseases and Syndromes

The number and locations of tender points help to define fibromyalgia according to the American College of Rheumatology; yet, there are many other symptoms and conditions that are associated with fibromyalgia. The most common associated symptoms are chronic fatigue, low-grade fever, swollen lymph nodes, anxiety, and depression. Other associated symptoms are:

- a weakened immune system with sore throats and swollen neck glands,
- headaches, migraines
- irritable bowel syndrome including symptoms of digestive complaints such as abdominal bloating, cramps, episodes of diarrhea and constipation, and problems of malabsorption;
- cold sensitivity, poor circulation, and heart palpitations,
- sleep difficulties,
- restless leg syndrome, lightheadedness, and dizziness,
- dry skin, dry eyes, and dry mouth.
- bladder infections in women,

- joint pain, tenderness, morning stiffness and burning sensations.
- numbness and tingling of hands and/or feet
- concentration problems and brain fog.

The chronic fatigue often associated with fibromyalgia makes some patients incapable of performing normal activities. Even minor exertion aggravates pain and creates additional episodes of fatigue, without a specific cause except lack of quality sleep. This fatigue is often described as feeling totally drained of energy. Many patients say that their arms and legs are so heavy they feel like concrete blocks. This fatigue also affects the cognitive ability in the brain to think clearly.

Headaches were common associated complaints in participants in the research project. One participant said that her head pain feels like "brain freeze", similar to the pain that we get when we eat ice cream too quickly. However, she had that feeling of pain constantly. There are many types of headaches, including migraines and sinus congestion pressure. Headaches have multiple causes, yet most can be relieved with increased circulation to the neck and head area, and by making sure the body is hydrated well.

Fibromyalgia is often associated with poor, non-restorative sleep. Patients with the disease wake up in the morning more exhausted than when they went to bed. Any type of poor sleep may precipitate fibromyalgia; on the other hand, the disease itself may lead to poor sleep. Since most patients with fibromyalgia have a poor sleep pattern, it is difficult to know which came first, the disease or the sleeping problem. One interesting research study, about lack of sleep, shows that normal people kept awake for several days develop trigger points similar to those found on patients with fibromyalgia.

Digestive disturbances are also associated factors in fibromyalgia syndrome. A common condition called 'Leaky Gut Syndrome' is related to malabsorption problems. When foods are not properly digested, and the lining of the intestines becomes weakened, the food particles leak through the wall of the intestine. This creates intestinal inflammation because the nutrients are not properly broken down and become toxic to the system. Symptoms such as bloating, flatulence, diarrhea and constipation are signs that there are digestive malabsorption problems.

The immune system is affected by a dysfunctional digestive system. Symptoms such as sinus congestion, sore throats, swollen glands, and lymph nodes are caused by bacterial imbalances in the intestines. Many of these symptoms and conditions become systemic; due to the way they disable the normal functions and activities of the patient.

[1] Campbell, SM, et.al. *Clinical Characteristics of Fibrositis, A Blinded Controlled Study of Symptoms and Tender Points*, Arthritis Rheum 1983;26:817-824

[2] Wolfe F. *The Clinical Syndrome of Fibrositis*, Am J Med 1986;8:7-13

[3] Wilke, W, *Fibromyalgia: Recognizing and addressing the multiple interrelated factors*. Postgraduate Med. 1996:100(1):153-170.

❧5❧

Part II

Causes of Fibromyalgia Symptoms

The causes of fibromyalgia are unknown; yet, researchers have several theories about what initiates or triggers the onset of the disorder. An increased level of chronic muscle tissue breakdown has been found to be one of the main reasons for the aching, pain, and fatigue. The onset may be gradual or sudden. Often symptoms may appear after a traumatic event or illness, or after a stressful episode. Traumatic experiences can cause injury to the nervous system sensors that make the muscles more hypersensitive to any reaction. This nervous system hypersensitivity can precipitate the tenderness on light touch often found in fibromyalgia patients. Fibromyalgia may also be associated with changes in the muscle metabolism, leading to decreased blood flow, fatigue, and diminished strength. Another factor that may cause fibromyalgia is a specific virus or bacteria, but no such infectious agent has been identified. No conclusive patterns have been identified to be responsible for fibromyalgia syndrome. A variety of metabolic conditions are probably the cause of the symptoms.

When the metabolic process malfunctions, congestion occurs in the fibrous tissues due to the lack of circulation from lack of energy. Our bodies need energy to complete every function, from thinking, breathing, fighting illness, and digesting food, to growing new cells. The energy used by the body to do every function is called adenosine triphosphate (ATP). In most healthy cells, the balances of substances needed to create ATP are carefully maintained. But in people diagnosed with fibromyalgia, these substances may become out of balance. Adenosine triphosphate is composed of an adenosine molecule attached to three phosphate molecules. These phosphate molecules are used to help to produce energy in the mitochondria, or energy centers of the cells, especially in the muscle and brain cells.

Research shows that fibromyalgia patients may also be deficient in certain minerals required for the synthesis of adenosine triphosphate (ATP), which include oxygen, magnesium, and phosphorus. The mitochondria in every cell need these minerals to produce ATP for energy within the cells. Deficiencies slow the metabolism and increase lactic acid formation. Lactic acid causes the soreness that occurs after exercising. When this lactic acid stays in the system, this increases the amount of muscle tissue breakdown that leads to the symptoms of fatigue, depression, and muscle pain. After pain, fatigue is the second most common symptom of fibromyalgia syndrome. Studies show that both chronic fatigue syndrome and fibromyalgia may have a common link in symptoms and the metabolic factors that can cause them to occur.

In the research study, the number of participants who listed an accident or trauma that triggered the fibromyalgia symptoms was 28 out of 50, or 56%. In some cases, accidents or traumas cause enough nervous system stress to initiate painful responses in the body. The effects of trauma stay in the body creating biochemical and nervous system changes. Unless the trauma is released, the stress continues to build up, creating chronic stress. Thirty percent of the fibromyalgia participants indicated that an accident, such as a car accident or fall brought on the symptoms. Some of the other initiating factors were colitis, cancer, surgery, scarlet fever, and emotional factors. In fact, 12% listed emotional trauma, such as divorce, abuse, or death of a loved one, as the initiating factor. When the fibromyalgia seems to be caused by an infection or another disease, it is the result of the infection not totally leaving the body and being retained in the lymph tissues.

In the following sections we will look deeper into causes of many chronic diseases, including fibromyalgia. First, we will look at the effect impaired digestion has on health. Then we will look at nervous system imbalances that cause pain and hypersensitivity. The next section is on stress and sleep disorders, including adrenal imbalances, fatigue, and emotional causes. Finally, we will look deeper into oxidative stress, and acid and alkaline imbalances. By learning about these topics you will understand the need for improved nutrition daily.

∝6∽

Impaired Digestion

On my first day of my natural healing course, the subject was digestion. We were taught, "85% of all diseases begin in the colon". As doctors of natural health, we were taught to look first for imbalances in the digestive system that could be the cause of symptoms in other parts of the body. After years of experience, I have found that in most cases this statement is definitely true. Even when there are symptoms in other parts of the body, such as chronic upper respiratory congestion or arthritic pain, it is often initiated by imbalances in the digestive tract. The health of our whole system can be determined by the foods we eat and how they are digested.

The digestive process begins in the mouth. When we chew food, we begin to break it down and digest it using the enzymes in the saliva. When the food gets to the stomach it needs to be broken down even more. The stomach needs to secrete enough hydrochloric acid to get the stomach enzymes activated. This can take up to 30 minutes to occur. When this process takes too long, indigestion happens. When heartburn occurs, it is actually due to the lack of hydrochloric acid in the stomach, which causes the food to ferment, building up gas in the stomach and esophagus, and producing pressure in the chest area. Only by getting the stomach to secrete its hydrochloric acid and enzymes effectively, will food be broken down. Taking antacids to slow or stop the secretion of hydrochloric acid inhibits the ability of the stomach to digest food properly. Antacids may help to prevent heartburn in the upper digestive tract from the mouth to the stomach, yet cause more problems in the lower digestive tract with undigested food.

When undigested food gets into the small intestine, it causes mucus to build up in the attempt to protect the lining of the intestinal wall. This mucus forms to counteract the bacteria created as the food ferments. In the small and large intestine there is supposed to be a high level of good bacteria. But with fermenting food, more toxic bacteria are created. The toxic bacteria overpower the good bacteria whenever there is undigested food in the intestinal tract. The toxic bacteria flourish when food sits too long and begins to putrefy or rot. If the undigested food is not removed quickly through the colon, toxic chemicals, called indicans, will form, and cause irritation to the lining of the digestive tract. As this irritation gets worse, the toxic chemicals are "leaked" through the intestine into the circulatory and lymph system. This condition is called "leaky gut syndrome", and has been linked to fibromyalgia as one of the associated syndromes. Actually, leaky gut syndrome is often the cause of many chronic disease patterns. You can prevent or reverse these disease patterns by making sure you digest food in the stomach effectively, and have enough good bacteria in the small intestine and colon for food to get broken down completely.

The gradual accumulation of toxic chemicals in the soft tissues is one of the causes of pain, especially in areas where we tend to hold stress, such as the neck, shoulders, and lower back. Any place where toxins build up in the tissues, the blood becomes thicker, slowing down circulation, and slowing down healing. Tender points can also develop due to conditions caused by a lack of oxygen getting into and being used by the cells. Insufficient oxygen in any cell of the body interferes with the healing process. The accumulation of toxic chemicals, lack of circulation, and the lack of oxygen, all lead to sluggishness in the lymph system. When the lymph fluid becomes stagnant, it causes the lymph nodes to swell and become sore. The pain in the tender points relate to this buildup of toxic lymph tissue in these areas. A natural consequence of too little oxygen is the build-up of lactic acid, causing soreness in these hypersensitive areas of tender points.

There are two principal ways that chemical toxins enter the body through the blood stream. They come in as a result of what is consumed, and what is breathed. At first the body will reject toxins. When we cough or sneeze, or when we vomit after eating contaminated foods, our bodies are trying to eliminate toxins. But over time, especially when these toxic chemicals are introduced into our bodies in minuscule amounts, the blood and organs get weakened, and the toxins build up in the tissues.

How do you know if you have digestive imbalances? You can know by the intensity of symptoms you have in the following areas:

Digestive symptoms - bad breath, gas, bloating, heartburn, constipation, diarrhea, foul odor to the stool, food allergies, hiatal hernia, and tired after meals.

Respiratory symptoms - sinus congestion, ear congestion, reoccurring bronchitis, and asthma.

Nervous system symptoms - loss of concentration or memory, anxiety, irritability, excessive worry, coordination problem, and depression.

Circulatory symptoms - headache or migraine, arthritis, cold hands and feet, low back pain.

Skin symptoms - body odor, eczema, psoriasis.

If you get tired after meals, you can check for toxic bacteria in the intestine by changing your diet. For three days eat nothing with sugar, including no fruit, no juice, no soft drinks, and no refined carbohydrates like bread or pasta. During the three days you can eat vegetables, plain yogurt, brown rice, water, and soy products. Notice if you feel better by looking at the change in your symptoms and energy level. If you feel better, it is demonstrating that fermenting food is producing toxic bacteria. These toxins are affecting the creation of your energy. There are a number of enzymes that are used to make energy that can become deactivated by these toxins, and therefore result in fatigue. Other circumstances that can deactivate these enzymes, in addition to sugar, include yeast imbalances in the small intestine, and environmental heavy metal toxicity, such as mercury and lead, and carbon monoxide pollution.

Malabsorption Urine Test

In addition to noticing your symptoms, you can also take a urine test to see the exact measurement of indicans present in your system. The Malabsorption Urine Test indicates elevated anaerobic bacteria activity in the small and large intestines. At elevated levels this test is an indicator of dysbiosis from intestinal toxemia and anaerobic bacteria and fungal growth.[4] When there is a bowel imbalance, nutrients cannot be absorbed as necessary. This test is also known as the Urinary

Indican Test where chloroform is mixed with the indican reagent and urine, and the results are observed after mixing thoroughly and waiting for the reaction to occur.[5] The color changes are on a scale of 0 to 4. 0 appearing as clear white, 1, 2, and 3, are various shades of blue getting darker with each higher number, and 4 appearing as black. This test reveals the absorption capacity of the digestive system. Fibromyalgia clients in the research study often complained of digestive disturbances that were related to this imbalance.

In the research study, the results showed that the fibromyalgia clients were more likely to have malabsorption problems. 72% of the fibromyalgia clients had some malabsorption imbalances compared to just 24% of the people in the control group. Also the average level of imbalance was much higher in the fibromyalgia group. There were three times more people in the fibromyalgia group with deep malabsorption problems than in the control group. This shows that impaired digestion can be measured, and definitely affects the symptoms of fibromyalgia.

The liver is the organ that has the greatest responsibility to keep the body clear of toxins. The liver uses minerals and enzymes to neutralize toxic chemicals. When neutralized toxic chemicals enter the blood, they can be eliminated easily through the colon or kidneys. The liver has two steps, or phases, to eliminate toxins from the system. In phase 1, the liver uses an enzyme to oxidize, or remove, toxic chemicals from the blood. In phase 2, the liver changes the toxic chemicals into a water-soluble state to be more easily removed by the body. When the phases of the liver detoxification system are not working efficiently, then any toxic chemicals created by undigested food will cause more stress on the liver. When the liver has continued to use up all the minerals to suppress the toxic chemicals, it will become congested. Then the liver cannot carry out its metabolic functions as efficiently. Once the liver is over 70% congested, toxic chemicals collect in the blood and eventually in the connective tissues.

The storage of toxic chemicals in tissue creates symptoms such as excess mucus, skin conditions, and either diarrhea or constipation. Again these symptoms are the body's response to these toxic chemicals and should not be suppressed. When the body is in a healthy state the chemical toxins can be released through the system more quickly. This is called an acute disease pattern. In this pattern, the toxins are released through the skin, or through the mucus membranes in the nose or throat. This is why we should not stop "cold" symptoms. They are often cleansing reactions trying to get toxins out of our system.

Once the body is weakened from a build up of congestion, it is best to take smaller steps in the cleansing process. This will assist in eliminating detoxifying reactions such as headaches and diarrhea. This weakened condition is called a chronic disease pattern. Most often the body develops a weakened chronic condition from suppressing the acute cleansing reactions we just discussed. When the acute reaction is suppressed, the toxic chemicals build up in the cells creating chronic symptoms from an increased toxic state. The vitality of the body is lessened and it becomes even more difficult to remove the toxins. The body begins to become fatigued and the weakened tissues degenerate from their normal function. This can be the beginning of autoimmune diseases or syndromes such as chronic fatigue syndrome or fibromyalgia.

What are effective ways to remove these chemical toxins from your system? First, make sure that your digestive system is working as effectively as possible. To activate the digestive juices, use fresh lemon juice in water. This will promote the proper digestion of food in the stomach. In addition to lemon in water, use a betaine hydrochloric acid supplement with stomach enzymes such as pepsin. The hydrochloric acid will help to digest the food more quickly in the stomach. Additional digestive enzyme supplementation will assist the small intestine to break the food into nutrients.

If constipation, diarrhea, or gas and bloating are a problem, the use of an herbal fiber supplement would be beneficial. Many herbs work as cleansers or gentle laxatives to remove toxic chemicals from the colon. The most common herbal fiber supplement is psyllium husks that absorb excess wastes in the small and large intestine. Psyllium needs to be consumed with a good quantity of water, otherwise the psyllium can become stuck in the colon if it is too dry for it to move through. Along with psyllium, herbs such as cascara sagrada and senna are used as gentle laxatives that stimulate the muscles of the colon to move wastes through more quickly. Intestinal gas is reduced with the use of peppermint, or other carminative herbs. Peppermints are served in restaurants after dinner to enhance digestion so that symptoms of gas or bloating are minimized. Another important type of herb to use to cleanse the colon is a moisturizer such as slippery elm or marshmallow. These herbs help keep the lining of the colon from becoming irritated. Additional herbs, such as dandelion, ginger, and yellow dock, are often included in herbal fiber cleansing to help the liver in the detoxification process.

When beginning to take herbal fiber supplements, start with one-quarter of the recommended dosage, and gradually increase the dosage every few days or every week. This will prevent cleansing reactions from toxins moving out of the system too quickly. After being on the recommended amount for one month, you can gradually decrease the dosage to a maintenance dose. An herbal fiber cleanse usually takes about three months to be effective. This three-month period includes the gradual build-up the first month, one month on the full dosage, and the gradually decrease the last month.

Normally, eighty-five percent of the bacteria in the colon are supposed to be the "good" or beneficial type of bacteria. Yet, in individuals with malabsorption problems, there is a definite increase in toxic bacteria. An imbalance of bacteria can also be caused by the consumption of sugar and processed food, the use of steroid medications and aspirin, and stress. Symptoms of lower bowel gas, bloating, constipation, skin problems, chronic upper respiratory congestion, and undigested food in the stool, all indicate an imbalance of bacteria in the colon.

To assist in rebalancing the bacteria in the colon certain foods or supplements containing acidophilus are used. Yogurt is the most common food containing live cultures of acidophilus. Most often we hear of using acidophilus to counter the effects of antibiotics in the system. It is best not to take acidophilus at the same time as antibiotics. Antibiotics are used to kill bacterial growth, including both beneficial bacteria and toxic bacteria. When you are taking antibiotics, let the medication do its job. Then, during the recovery process the acidophilus can be used. Acidophilus is a supplement that is found in the refrigerated section of health food stores. Acidophilus has an antibacterial and antifungal effect, lowers cholesterol, helps with the absorption of nutrients, and detoxifies the colon of toxic bacteria.

The digestive system needs to be functioning as effectively as possible at all times. Using herbs, acidophilus, and changing the diet, are all helpful, but making sure the toxic chemicals are moved out of the body, as quickly as possible, is most important. "The solution to pollution is dilution" is a phrase used to remind us to drink plenty of water every day. Keep the tissues hydrated so that toxic chemicals can be flushed out, before congestion occurs. One of the major causes of constipation, skin rashes, asthma and other signs of toxin build-up is a lack of adequate water getting into the tissues. Later we will discuss the importance of water in making sure the body is hydrated enough to keep toxins out of the system and nutrients in the system.

[4] Curzon G., and Walsh J., "*Value of Measuring Urinary Indican Excre*tion:, Gut 7:711, 1966.

[5] Hamilton, J.D., et.al., "*Assessment and Significance of Bacterial Overgrowth in the Small Bowel*", QJ Med, 39 (154):265-285, April 1970

❧7❧

Hypersensitivity to Pain

The pain of fibromyalgia can vary between deep muscular aching, throbbing, burning, shooting and stabbing pains. Often, the pain and stiffness are worse in the morning. Once simple movement gets circulation to the muscles the pain may decrease. Often, pain may be worse in the muscle groups that are used repetitively. The health of the nervous system can also affect the pain response in the body. Neuropathy is a term used to describe nerve disease or injury. The most common type of neuropathy is a pinched nerve. The deep spinal muscles cause most of the nerves to feel pinched. The term myofascial dysfunction describes muscle and tendon pain with neuropathy. "Myo" refers to muscle, and "fascia" refers to the connective tissue of muscle and tendon. Together, myofascial pain and neuropathy affect muscle dysfunction that leads to various patterns of acute or chronic pain.

An important principle in understanding the cause of pain is Cannon's Law. Walter Cannon and Arthur Rosenbleuth researched the chemical mechanisms of nerve impulse transmission in the 1940's, and found that any tissue that becomes denervated becomes supersensitive. Denervated tissue means that the nerves in that tissue do not send nerve impulses effectively. Cannon's Law specifically stated is: "When a unit is destroyed in a series of efferent neurons, an increased irritability to chemical agents develops in the isolated structures, the effect being maximal in the part directly denervated."[6]   In other words, when a nerve link to a part of the body fails, that part of the body becomes highly irritable and electrically sensitive. This super sensitivity of the tissues can occur in many parts of the body including the skeletal muscle, smooth muscle, spinal neurons, sympathetic nerve endings, adrenal glands, and even brain cells. External temperature and barometric changes can also affect the pressure of cellular fluids on the nervous system. This is another reason fibromyalgia patients have specific tender points of pain, and are often sensitive to changes in weather.

Muscle spasms and chronic contraction of muscle fibers can be caused by this super sensitivity in the nervous system tissue. These spasms do not go away until the nerve function is restored. This explains why a person with a low back pinched nerve has trouble with hamstring tightness and cannot bend over. As muscles remain persistently spastic or in a contracted position, they will eventually shorten and become tight causing abnormal joint movement and compression. This will lead to abnormal wear points in the joints and cause pain in the connective tissues.

A build-up of toxins in the tissues causes these muscle spasms, stiffness and hypersensitivity. There are a couple remedies to reverse these muscle and nervous system imbalances. One is drinking enough water to improve circulation in the tissues. The other is to use essential fatty acids, such as evening primrose oil or borage oil, to increase the flexibility of the cells and transmit nerve impulses efficiently. We will look at the specific benefits and uses of essential fatty acids in the section on nutritional supplements.

Substance P, a polypeptide made of several amino acids bonded together, is made naturally in the body and is stored in the nervous system and intestines. The function of Substance P is to stimulate the expansion and contraction of smooth muscles in the intestines and in other places. It also has an effect in the pain response recognized by the nervous system. Substance P is released in response to physical injury in muscles and tissues, and is abundantly found in fibromyalgia patients. It stimulates the release of histamine that causes tissue swelling, smooth muscle contraction, and pain transmission. A study done at the Medical College of Wisconsin in Milwaukee used capsaicin to reduce the sensation of pain and reduce excess reserves of Substance P. Capsaicin is a phytochemical found in cayenne pepper, and is used in many pain-relieving creams. The four-week study had 45 people using capsaicin cream (0.025%), and found that there was a significant decrease in the areas where the cream was applied.[7]

Other herbs that are commonly used to reduce pain in the muscles are ginger, turmeric and boswellia. These herbs improve the circulation and help the liver detoxify. Ginger and turmeric are known as digestive herbs and spices that are used to increase circulation and reduce inflammation. Boswellia is an Ayurvedic herb that nourishes the soft tissues by improving blood supply to the muscles to help reduce stiffness. There are some herbal formulas on the market that combine these three herbs together. Begin with just a couple tablets or capsules a day, and increase gradually to at least 3 capsules or tablets three times per day. With the use of liquid herbal extracts, 30 drops is equivalent to 3 capsules. Since herbs are made from a whole plant they often have more than one effect in the body, compared to the single purpose of a prescription drug.

It is important that you begin taking any herb slowly to avoid any reaction with other substances you may be taking. It is recommended with any herb, or vitamin and mineral formula, to take them regularly for 6 days a week, and then do not take them on the seventh day. This allows your body the chance to integrate the action of the herb or supplement on its own. After 3 months, evaluate the effectiveness of the herbal supplement. This should give your system time to see the benefits of the herb. When using ginger, turmeric, and boswellia, it is best to increase the dosage to the maximum allowed for at least a couple of weeks to get the full effect of the herb and then reduce the amount to a maintenance dose. Herbs are concentrated plant substances that assist the body in supporting the natural healing response. So when you find an herb or herbal combination that works well for you, remember the name of it. Since everyone is different, specific herbs will help specific people, and often you will be able to go back to that herb to help you stay healthy.

---

[6] Rosenblueth, A. and Cannon, W.B., *The Supersensitivity of Denervated Structures. A Law of Denervation",* MacMillan, Neuva, NY, 1949.

[7] McCarty, Daniel J. et.al. *Treatment of Pain Due to Fibromyalgia with Topical Capsaicin: A Plot,* Seminars in Arthritis and Rheumatism, 23:6 Suppl 3, 41-47.

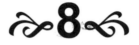

Stress Factors and Sleep Disturbances

Everyday we are affected by the environment we live in. The way we respond to this environment instigates the stresses in our lives. Our relationships, our work environment, our diet and exercise program, and our habits, both good and bad, all are stressful to our health as regulated by our adrenal glands. All illnesses are stressful. Chronic worries, such as financial or relationship problems, subject the body to stress. For many people taking a test is very stressful. Driving can also be very stressful. Stress, in fact, is a major killer of many people.

One of the questions on the fibromyalgia research questionnaire asked what triggers the fibromyalgia pain. The number that listed stress as making the pains worse was 22 out of 50. Since stress includes many potential causes, and the parameters of stress are vague, stress as a cause of the pain is difficult to measure. Secondary to stress, exertion was the next factor to make the pain worse. Other factors that also have an effect, according to the research participants, were lack of sleep, weather, inactivity, diet and fatigue. It was interesting to note that too much exertion or physical labor causes the pain to get worse, and yet, total rest or inactivity also creates stiffness that inflated the pain. Morning stiffness is a common complaint; yet, once movement begins, the pain tends to subside. Weather, especially cold, damp weather, or cold water also increase the pain.

Another question on the questionnaire asked what the participants do to relieve pain. In this case, the most common answer was to take some type of pain pills (32%), such as Motrin or Tylenol. The second and third answers were to stretch or exercise (24%), and to get a massage (22%). Other common ways to reduce pain were to take a hot shower or use a hot tub (20%), rest (16%), or apply hot (14%), or cold packs (12%). A few people also used vitamin and mineral supplementation, sleep, visualization, acupuncture, and physical therapy for pain reduction.

One of the most common symptoms of fibromyalgia is sleep disturbance due to the chronic pain. These sleep problems can come from anxiety, which causes more muscle pain, and causes more sleep problems. Chronic pain will disrupt normal sleep cycles by acting as a stimulant, which will then affect sleeping ability even more. Often medications and supplements that block pain, or reduce anxiety can help create more restful sleep.

Remembering the stresses of the day often causes trouble falling asleep. The body remains tense and the adrenaline keeps flowing as long as thoughts and activities related to stress are maintained. For at least one hour before going to bed, it is far more beneficial to engage in a quiet activity, relax in a warm bath, or meditate, than it is to watch television or do something mentally demanding. It is recommended to get between 8 and 10 hours of sleep regularly.

Sleep restores neurotransmitters. Tryptophan is an amino acid neurotransmitter that helps produce serotonin, which fights depression and helps promote sleep. Tryptophan is found in turkey, milk, lentils, soybeans, and tuna. Eating those foods before sleep will help to promote serotonin production. To assist daily neurotransmitter restoration it is best to get to bed by 10 p.m. Your nervous system tends to get a burst of energy between 10 p.m. and midnight if you are still awake, using more neurotransmitters to function.

In order for your body to operate efficiently, it must synthesize chemical energy for it's various organs, cells and processes. There are approximately 30 different kinds of energy that need to be synthesized. If one or more of these become impaired, you begin to feel tired. If you have impaired energy synthesis, you will need lots of sleep, 8 to 11 hours per day, to create energy. If you find that you feel worse during the day if you get less than 8 hours sleep, this may be due to depleted energy.

Low blood sugar promotes the release of cortisone and adrenaline from the adrenals, and increases liver function. If the blood sugar fluctuates during the evening, it can cause the adrenals to become more stressed and sleep will be disturbed. Sleep disturbances are caused by many factors including the functioning of the adrenals, pancreas, and other endocrine glands. The sleep problems related to fibromyalgia syndrome are brought about by a variety of causes, and each person must look at their overall symptoms to discover how they can individually be helped.

❧9❧

Adrenal Stress and Fatigue

The adrenal glands are two organs that sit on top of each kidney. They are shaped like small pyramids and are just a bit smaller than your palms. They help us respond to stresses in our lives. Your adrenals work with the pituitary and the hypothalamus to secrete hormones to keep the effects of stress in check in the glandular system. The adrenal glands produce specific hormones in response to different levels of stress. The inner part of your adrenal glands, called the adrenal medulla, secrete adrenalin and noradrenalin. These hormones are increased when you experience acute stress such as anger and fear. They are the hormones that help you gain energy for quick responses like running, lifting or fighting. These hormones cause an immediate rush of ATP that is stored in the muscles. This is the adrenal response that can make you extraordinarily strong for a short period of time.

The adrenal cortex, on the outside portion of the adrenal gland, responds to chronic stresses. The adrenal cortex manufactures steroid hormones including cortisone, hydrocortisone, testosterone, estrogen, DHEA, cholesterol, pregnenolone, aldosterone, and progesterone. The adrenals are the major steroid factories of the body. The three hormones made only in the adrenal cortex are cortisone, hydrocortisone, and aldosterone. Aldosterone works together with the kidneys to regulate the mineral balance in the body. The proper balance of minerals is critically important in a healthy stress response. Cortisone and hydrocortisone help regulate the level of glucose in the body by converting protein to glucose.

Under normal conditions, the adrenal glands have enough cortisone, hydrocortisone, and aldosterone to respond when there is stress and more energy is needed. When these hormones are secreted, more energy is released, and the problem is handled, then our physiology returns to a relaxed condition. However, the adrenal glands can only take so much stress. When this level of adrenal stress is surpassed, the adrenals respond as well as they can — by making all the cortisone, hydrocortisone, and aldosterone that they can, releasing them, then make some more, release them, and so on. At first this repetitive response creates adrenal stress, causing too much cortisol and aldosterone in the system. Your body will use up minerals quickly, and weight gain will occur more easily as the increased cortisol levels cause insulin resistance.

Adrenal stress comes from prolonged release of adrenaline hormones, a chronic elevation of heart rate and muscle tension, and a decrease in blood flow to organs. In addition, there is an increase in the retention of sodium, water and calcium, and a thickening of the blood. Adrenal stress will deplete minerals, reduce immune system health, and increases fat storage from increased cortisol build-up. When cortisol is increased it brings on symptoms of fatigue, irritability, hypoglycemia, night sweats, sugar cravings, binge eating and mental confusion.

Eventually, the adrenals become fatigued due to chronic stress, lack of sufficient vitamins and minerals, not enough sleep, lack of exercise, poor bowel function or hypoglycemia. As adrenal stress continues, the adrenals actually become more fatigued, which causes changes in mood, weakness from a decrease in the ability to create energy effectively, more depressive and confused thinking and increased susceptibility to allergies.

Eventually, you become so tired that you just "cannot take it any more." You rest for a few days and feel well enough to go again, but then the cycle repeats itself. After a few months or years of chronic stress the adrenal glands become weak. Even after resting they are unable to respond to stress in a normal manner. The most common clinical manifestation of this condition is chronic fatigue. Other signs of weak adrenal function include overeating and weight gain especially in the abdominal area. When the adrenals are completely nonfunctional, the result is weight loss, excessive loss of salt from the kidneys and abnormally low blood pressure. This condition is called Addison's disease and is most commonly seen in females. Only by strengthening the adrenals through diet, nutritional supplements and emotional stress reduction exercises will the adrenal fatigue improve.

In the presence of exhausted adrenals, the immune system function is seriously weakened. This makes people more susceptible to a variety of infections. Always look for weak adrenal or thyroid glands when you tend to get "everything that is going around", since the immune system is compromised. For example, the incidence of autoimmune disease goes up in the presence of weak adrenals. When the adrenals become fatigued, the immune system is allowed to attack certain cells of the body as if they were foreign invaders.

Anyone who becomes exhausted after stress, and remains exhausted, should have his or her adrenals tested. This is especially true for people who become exhausted for days after even slight exertion. By having the adrenals tested you can see the level of adrenal stress or fatigue, and can begin taking supplements to improve the imbalance. A relaxing massage helps to reduce stress, as well as other relaxation techniques such as meditation, and both will gradually improve adrenal function.

Adrenal Stress Test

The Adrenal Stress Test is a urine test that determines levels of adrenal stress or adrenal fatigue, levels of cortisol and chlorides in the urine, degree of energy output, and potential magnesium, potassium and calcium deficiency. The adrenal glands play an important role in regulating the body's adaptation to stress. The "fight and flight" mode of the adrenal glands occurs when the sympathetic nervous system responses to acute stress.

The Adrenal Stress Test measures the chloride displacement into the urine. The Adrenal Stress number is determined by counting the number of silver nitrate drops added to urine, and a potassium chromate indicator solution, before a reaction occurs. When a reaction occurs with 1 to 13 drops of silver nitrate, it indicates adrenal stress, with increased cortisol, sodium and chlorides in the system, and where the body is using up minerals quickly to defend this stressed state. Adrenal stress is a stage of adrenal function where there is sustained activation of the sympathetic nervous system, and the blood sugar tends to become elevated. When a reaction occurs with 14 to 25 drops of silver nitrate drops, it indicates a normal adrenal response.

When over 25 drops is needed to create a
reaction, it is an indication of adrenal fatigue, with low
levels of chlorides, sodium and cortisol, and very low
readings of excess minerals are found in the urine.[8]
Adrenal fatigue includes symptoms of extreme fatigue,
hypoglycemia, food sensitivities, headaches, low blood
pressure, and lowered concentration ability. These
readings are explained in the following charts.

Number of Silver Nitrate Drops	Reaction Results
1 to 13 drops	Adrenal Stress
14 to 25 drops	Normal Adrenal
Over 25 drops	Adrenal Fatigue

In the research study, the fibromyalgia group
had a greater incidence of both adrenal stress and
adrenal fatigue than the people in the control group.
Twenty-eight percent of people in the fibromyalgia
group had readings of adrenal stress, compared to 20%
in the control group. On the other side, 28% of people in
the fibromyalgia group had readings of adrenal fatigue
compared to 22% in the control group. Overall, it is a
difference of 56% of people with adrenal imbalance in
the fibromyalgia group compared to 42% in the control
group. The following chart shows the number of
participants with abnormal readings in the Adrenal
Stress Test from the fibromyalgia study.

	Fibromyalgia Group	Control Group	Difference
Adrenal Stress	28%	20%	8%
Adrenal Fatigue	28%	22%	6%
Totals	56%	42%	14%

While this does not show a great deal of difference in the adrenal stress and adrenal fatigue reading for fibromyalgia clients compared to the control group, it does show that increased stress can cause excessive symptoms.

---

[8] Bray, W.E., *"Clinical Laboratory Methods"*, St. Louis: C.V. Mosby Company, 1957:79-80.

❧10❦

Emotions and Health

Fibromyalgia has a strong emotional element. Twelve percent of the participants in the research study believe that an emotional trauma was the initial cause of their fibromyalgia. More than 50% of the participants believe that stress from their work or personal life makes the fibromyalgia pain worse. The emotions from the initiating trauma or everyday stress become trapped in the muscle tissues, and when held for a period of time constricts the muscles. Some of the common emotions that have been related to fibromyalgia are feelings of resentment and hopelessness from work or family stress, or from childhood memories.

Emotions can be held in the body and create physical imbalances. Any chronic emotion such as fear, anger, hostility or sadness will cause the adrenal glands to secrete cortisol. When cortisol is elevated for any length of time it will affect the behavior of certain organs. Hardening of the arteries and cancer are two examples of major causes of death that can be related to increased cortisol levels. Also, obesity is another problem related to excess cortisol levels. Excessive cortisol can cause gradual weight gain, especially in the abdominal area.

The immune system does require adequate levels of cortisol to function properly. This means that we need a certain amount of stress in our lives as stimulation for us to function effectively. Of course what constitutes an adequate level of stress varies from person to person. Excessive cortisol can speed up the immune system dangerously causing adrenal stress. For example, if you feel anger, yet you ignore it, soon you will find an elevation of anger in many other areas of your life. Eventually you'll believe that everyone is against you. Your body continues to secrete cortisol to make immune antibody cells to counteract all this pent up emotion. You will become more prone to chronic fatigue, and chronic colds or immune weakness. Ultimately, you will have so many excess antibodies they will turn against each other causing autoimmune diseases.

Alternatively, your body can also become so tired of these excess emotions that you will be physically and emotionally exhausted of this struggle. Then your body will stop producing cortisol and immune cells. As these levels decrease, the body becomes chronically depressed, and adrenal fatigue develops. The body's minerals become exhausted from constantly trying to fight these emotions, and the immune system becomes worn out. In this state, susceptibility to infections, and sensitivities to environmental chemicals increase, while the lack of necessary energy to heal well, is not available.

In Chinese medicine, certain emotions are related to certain organs. Chinese medicine also links organs into five elements called Fire, Earth, Metal, Water and Wood. For example the heart is equated with the fire element and its associated emotions are joy and happiness. The spleen and stomach are associated with the earth element, and with the emotions of anxiety and worry. Anxious thoughts create immune system stress by affecting the spleen. The lungs and large intestine are equated with the metal element, and are associated with grief and conflict. The kidney and bladder are coupled in the water element, and emotionally are related to insecurity and restlessness. The liver and gall bladder are related to the wood element, and emotionally associated with anger and resentment. For example when anger becomes chronic, the liver physically enlarges and the many functions of the liver are affected. Recognizing your reoccurring emotions will enable you to identify the type of stress you may be inflicting on your organs.

Specifically, according to Chinese Medicine, the symptoms of fibromyalgia have been linked most often to liver, gallbladder, and spleen meridian imbalances. The liver meridian stores and cleanses the blood, maintains the flow of energy, controls the contractility and flexibility of the muscles, ligaments and tendons. When the liver energy is deficient, dryness occurs in the skin and tendons, and smooth flow of blood in the body is constricted. Also liver imbalances bring on symptoms of frustration, irritability, and feeling stuck, commonly produce an emotional state of constant resentment, with repressed anger or depression.

The gallbladder meridian is the source of courage and initiative, and is responsible for decision-making. Physically, the gallbladder meridian controls circulation of the energy that protects and nourishes the cells, and when out of balance weakens the ligaments and tendons. Symptoms of insomnia, wandering pains, weakness in the legs, and chest and side pains are caused by gallbladder weakness.

The spleen meridian governs digestion, and imbalances manifest in the muscles. The spleen meridian also relates to feelings of stability, including feeling centered and balanced. The excessive use of the mind tends to weaken the spleen meridian energy flow. This includes excess emotional worry, or anxiety about the future. Imbalance in the spleen meridian energy flow manifests as morning fatigue, craving for sweets, nausea, flatulence, loose stools, pale lips, swelling of the abdomen, and muscular weakness.

Emotions and your mental state may not seem important, and may be easy to ignore in your daily life. Yet, research has shown that it takes 6 hours for your immune system to recover from a quick negative emotional experience. On the other hand, when we have an encouraging emotional experience, there is an immediate increase in beneficial chemicals that have a positive effect on the immune system. For example, when we feel loved or appreciated and are reminded of it, nourishing chemicals are released into our immune system. Also, when we make positive statements, instead of negative statements, our own immune system is enhanced. Even our thoughts, whether positive or negative, will have an effect on our immune system. Having a critical temperament towards yourself and others will create more immune system problems than for those who have a positive temperament. Sometimes we are more critical of ourselves than we are of others. Remember to always treat others like you would want to be treated, and treat yourself like you want others to treat you.

The following is a story demonstrating how unresolved emotions can cause physical pain.

A few years ago, a relative called me with constant low back pain that began after being out of town for the weekend. She went to her medical doctor and he could not find anything that could be causing it. Medication did not help. Then she when to a chiropractor, and his treatment made the pain worse. Eventually, she called me to send her a homeopathic remedy to relieve the pain. I found a remedy that matched her physical symptoms. She took a few doses of the remedy the next day, and her pain went away. While talking about the quick relief from pain, I asked what, if anything, happened in her life just before this pain started. She remembered that just a couple days before the pain began, she had had an argument with her husband. This argument was not resolved before she went out of town.

This story is an example of emotional constipation, when low back pain comes from not letting go of conflict. She was physically holding onto this conflict in her lower back, which according to Chinese Medicine theory is a common place to hold unresolved issues. Homeopathic remedies work on physical and emotional symptoms, and often help resolve this type of emotional difficulty along with physical symptoms. Homeopathic remedies that are commonly used for fibromyalgia, to relieve both physical and emotional pain, are discussed later under the section on designing your own program.

❧11❧

Oxidative Stress

Smoke from burning wood, or when apples turn brown when they are cut open, are visual effects of oxidation. Oxidation, or too much oxygen, can cause the human body to degenerate, or age more quickly than usual, just as iron rusts as it breaks down. Oxygen is needed for life. Yet, too much oxygen causes oxidative stress, which in turn causes chronic degenerative diseases, because it causes the human body to essentially rust on the inside. An understanding of this oxidative process is important to maintaining health, and protecting the body from its own destruction.

What causes oxidative stress? It is caused by too many free radicals in the tissues of the body. Free radicals are unstable molecules looking to steal an electron from a healthy molecule. They are made of oxygen molecules that have at least one open electron in their outer shell. This open electron creates an electrical charge. To balance this charge, the free radicals attempt to get an electron from any molecule or substance in the vicinity. They have such aggressive movement that they chemically create bursts of light within the body. If these free radicals are not neutralized rapidly, they may create more free radicals or cause damage to blood vessel walls, cell walls, and even the DNA of the cell.

Our bodies are literally under attack potentially every minute by free radicals.

Free radicals target weaker areas of the body and determine what type of degenerative disease will develop. Some scientists believe each person has certain areas in their body that are genetically predisposed to oxidative stress, which may explain genetic-type traits when it comes to degenerative diseases. Every day in the energy center of each cell called the mitochondria, some oxidation occurs in the normal process of metabolism Antioxidants are the best defenses against the attack of free radicals. Antioxidants bind with the extra electron in the free radical and render the free radical harmless. As long as there are adequate amounts of antioxidants in the body to handle the free radicals produced within the cell, there is no damage to the surrounding tissues.

Metabolism produces many free radicals as waste products. In health, the body can neutralize and clear these chemicals. Yet, in illness, free radicals are produced in such large quantities that the body cannot neutralize them. Excess free radicals accumulate and cause oxidative stress and a build up of metabolic toxins. The most common symptoms of metabolic toxins are digestive distress, like bloating, diarrhea, and abdominal pain. More symptoms of metabolic oxidative stress are shortness of breath, fatigue after eating, and obesity. Metabolic toxins become worse once oxygen metabolism becomes dysfunctional, slowing down the healing process.

Many factors increase the amount of free radicals in the body. Excessive stress, excessive exercise, chemicals in our air, food and water, cigarette smoke, microwave foods, medications and radiation, saturated fats, and hydrogenated fats from processed foods, are all factors that cause free radicals. Margarine, made from hydrogenated fats, causes more free radicals to build up in the arteries, than butter. Butter has saturated fats, but the trans fats created from hydrogenated fats cannot be broken down by the metabolism, and live in the body as free radicals.

Stress is a fact of life, and mild or moderate stress only increases free radicals a small amount. Yet with severe emotional stress, free radical production goes up exponentially and can cause significant oxidative stress. Excessive exercise can be a cause of oxidative stress. When exercise is moderate, the production of free radicals increases, but not significantly. However, when exercise is excessive, the production of free radicals goes up exponentially, due to lactic acid buildup. Athletes who compete regularly should be sure to get adequate levels of antioxidants regularly to compensate for their exercise regimen.

There are many more chemicals and pollutants in air, food, and water, and more people are exposed to them than ever before. These chemical toxins include pesticides, fungicides, herbicides, industrial pollutants, toxic metal compounds, and synthetic hormones. The toxic burden of chemicals has increased markedly in the last fifty years. The effects of man-made chemicals are seen most often in the body as skin disorders, allergies, headaches, or lymph congestion that is chronic.

In large cities many people can smell the environmental chemicals. And in farming communities the smell of fertilizers and pesticides fill the air. The Environmental Protection Agency states that there are well over 70,000 chemicals being used commercially in the United States. Many of these are used in the production of our food, and many end up in our water supply. In 1999, over 50 contaminants are regularly monitored in municipal drinking water.[9] All of these chemicals and pollutants that enter the body must be handled in some way. Some are broken down and excreted, and others are stored as toxins, especially in our fat. All of these toxins significantly increase the amount of free radicals that the body produces. One of the greatest causes of oxidative stress is smoke from cigarettes. Many clinical studies have shown cigarette smoke causes tremendous production of excessive free radicals. There is also significant production of free radicals associated with secondary smoke. Again, the body will have to use the available antioxidants to reduce the free radicals from these pollutants.

Oxidative stress also comes from microbes such as yeasts, imbalanced bacteria, overactive viruses, and parasites produced even in healthy bodies. Those microbes multiply rapidly in the bowel and blood when the body has to manage other toxins from pesticides, pollutants, antibiotic overuse or sugar overload. When the level of microbes is increased, the common symptoms are chronic nasal congestion, sore throat and coughing, or chronic fatigue. All excess levels of microbes cause an increase in oxidative stress in the body that antioxidants and other nutrients have to control.

The effects of all these toxins and free radicals build up in the body causing chronic sluggish blood flow and stagnant lymph circulation. Stiffness and pain are the most common symptoms that come from this decrease circulation. Proteins in the circulating blood become more solid and form small clots when exposed to excessive oxidative stress factors. When these proteins become dense there is a decrease of blood flow causing the congestion in the tender points. As we improve our health, the effects of oxidative stress and these symptoms can be reduced.

Microwaved Food

Microwaved food has become a daily convenience. Though the food still looks good, after it is microwaved many of the beneficial qualities are lost. Using microwaves in cooking can deplete foods of their nutrients. Then when microwaved food is consumed, it can cause pathological changes in your body. Microwaves are high-frequency electromagnetic waves that alternate in positive and negative directions, causing vibration of food molecules up to 2.5 billion times per second. This creates friction and heat, changing the chemical composition of foods and liquids. The food becomes altered so much that our digestive system has trouble breaking it down into usable nutrients.

For example, in the April 1992, the *Journal of American Pediatrics* reported that microwaving breast milk, to warm it up, destroyed 98% of its immunoglobulin-A antibodies, necessary for strengthening the immune system of the infant, and 96% of enzyme activity that inhibits bacterial growth. In a German study in 1994, the blood measurements of 8 participants who were fed only baked foods were compared to the blood measurement of 8 other participants who ate only microwaved foods. During the two-month study, blood tests were performed three times per day to measure nutrient and bacterial levels. The blood measurements of the subjects who ate the microwave food were lower in hemoglobin, or red blood cells. Lowered hemoglobin can lead to anemia and thyroid imbalances. The white blood cell count was increased in those who ate microwaved vegetables. This increased white blood cell count indicated that the body was responding to the microwaved cooked food as an infectious agent. Blood measurements also noted that the level of "bad" cholesterol rose significantly after the consumption of microwaved vegetables.

While all heating methods have an effect on the level of nutrients, microwaving foods appears to produce the greatest losses. Since we eat foods to nourish our bodies, we should daily consider what types of foods we are eating. Continuously eating foods cooked in a microwave will gradually increase the number of toxins in our systems. Eventually, the instinctive healing process we all have within us will become out of balance.

Bio-Chemical Testing for Oxidative Stress

Different bio-chemical tests using urine are available to show results of oxidative stress on the body. The first test is the Free Radical Test, and is also called an anti-aging profile, since it shows the level of stress on the body caused by free radical activity. Aging occurs more quickly when our bodies have to deal with environmental stress in the form of microbes, chemicals and metabolic imbalances.

Free Radical Test

The Free Radical Test is a urine test that measures the level of free radical activity in the cells. When the rate of biochemical reactions in the intercellular fluid increases, there is a greater electron potential in the urine. By using an ampoule with malondialdehyde as the reagent, a measure of lipid peroxidation in the urine is calculated. The amount of lipid peroxidation relates to the level of tissue breakdown, which is relative to the amount of free radicals in the metabolism.[10] The level of color change from clear to dark pink after 5 minutes is evaluated. Too many free radicals over a period of time lead to chronic disease and faster aging. Free radical damage comes from oxidative stress caused by heavy metals and petrochemicals in the environment and in our foods, over-the-counter and prescription drugs, cooked oils and fats, radiation, viruses, yeast, and bacteria, and emotional stress. This test shows if you are getting enough antioxidants in your diet and supplementation program. Without adequate amounts of antioxidants, free radicals build up and oxidative stress reactions show in this Free Radical test.

In the research project this free radical test was done for both the fibromyalgia and control group. When the color of the urine changed to a light pink color in the vial, it indicated low free radical activity, and was measured as a one (1). When the color of the urine changed to a medium pink, it was an indication of medium free radical activity, and was recorded as a two (2). When the color changed to a bright pink, it indicated a high level of free radical activity, and was recorded as a three (3). The ideal reading is a one since everyone has some level of free radicals in their system at all times. The average of all readings for the fibromyalgia group was 2.32 compared the control group reading of 1.93. This indicates that there was a greater tendency for oxidative stress from free radical activity found in people who have fibromyalgia

Vitamin C Test

Vitamin C is essential for the production of connective tissue, and for support of the bones, blood vessels, joints, organs, muscles, eyes, teeth and skin. It also helps to create antibodies and white blood cells, to protect the mucus membranes of the body, improve stability of vitamin E, and improve the transport of iron into cells. The vitamin C test mixes dichlorolindophenol with drops of urine to see how it reacts with the ascorbic acid in the urine. A normal response is indicated when 5 or less drops of urine are needed to change the color of the dichlorolindophenol from blue to clear. A deficiency of ascorbic acid is indicated with more than 5 drops of urine added to change the color.[11] When vitamin C foods are consumed regularly, or effective vitamin C supplementation is used, the number of drops of urine needed to change the color decreases, depending on the amount of ascorbic acid in the urine.

The bio-chemical research test results for this Vitamin C test showed a decreased level of vitamin C in the fibromyalgia group. Ideally, the number of drops needed to create a reaction, showing sufficient vitamin C, is 5 drops or less. The control group needed an average of 6.72 drops to create a reaction, while the fibromyalgia group needed an average of 9.32 drops to create the reaction. This shows that there is a greater deficiency in vitamin C, the most common antioxidant, in people who have fibromyalgia.

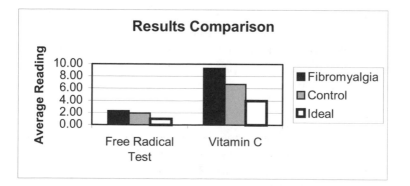

---

[9] Environmental Protection Agency,
www.epa.gov/ogwow/ccl/cclfs/html

[10] Draper H.H., *"Urinary Malondialdehyde as an Indicator of Lipid Peroxidation in the Diet and in the Tissues,"* Lipids 19(11):836-843, November 1984

[11] Saracci R., *"Quick Assessment of Vitamin C Status."* Lancet 1(7957); 490-491, Feb. 1976.

ᘓ12ᘗ

PH Levels and Acidity

All of the cells, organs and fluids in the body have their own ideal pH values in order to operate at peak performance. When the pH is higher or lower than the ideal level, the cells become stressed. Then these cells cannot utilize the nutrients they need, and cannot eliminate wastes efficiently, until the proper pH is restored. Testing the pH on a regular basis can easily monitor the pH levels.

Cell pH refers to the degree of acidity or alkalinity of the body's blood or other fluids. The number of hydrogen ions is calculated by measuring the pH levels in blood, saliva, and urine. Simply, the term pH means "potential hydrogen", and represents a scale for the relative alkalinity or acidity of a solution. The scale begins at 0.0 with a measure of the pH of sulphuric acid, and ends at 14.0 with the pH of pure calcium. The midpoint at 7.0 is a neutral reading. A number less than 7.0 pH indicates a more acid solution, and a number greater than 7.0 pH indicates a more alkaline solution. These numbers refer to how many hydrogen ions are present in the solution compared to a standard solution.

We are exposed to many types of acid and base substances that we use or consume everyday. Base substances taste bitter, and feel slippery or soapy. Some examples of base substances are soaps and detergents. Base substances produce hydroxyl (OH·) ions in liquid solutions. Acid substances produce hydrogen (H⁺) ions in liquids. Some examples of acid substances are citric acid found in fruits and vegetables, ascorbic acid found in fruits, vinegar, carbonic acid in soft drinks, and lactic acid found in buttermilk. Acid substances taste sour. In fact, the word "acid" comes from the Latin word *acere*, which means 'sour'. Acid liquid solutions conduct electric current, which makes them electrolytes, and react with bases to form salts and water.

Overview of pH Readings		
	$0.0 \Longleftarrow$ 7.0 pH $\Longrightarrow 14.0$	
PH:	Low	High
Reading:	Acid	Alkaline
Current:	Increased	Decreased
Resistance:	Low	High
Reactions Happen:		
	Too Fast	Too Slow

The pH values are on a logarithmic scale, indicating a ten-fold difference between each unit. For example, a pH of 6.0 is ten times more acid than a pH of 7.0, yet a pH of 5.0 is 100 times more acid then a pH of 7.0. Most pH readings for urine and saliva variations are read on a tenths scale, since just a few tenths of a point can indicate a significant difference between ideal health and illness. The pH reading is a measurement of the resistance of your tissues to electrical energy. As the pH moves lower than 7.0, the current flow increases through the solution since the resistance is lower. In this case, digestive enzymes and minerals, especially calcium, move through the system too quickly to be absorbed effectively. When the pH is above 7.0, there is a decrease in the potential current flow and an increase in resistance. When the resistance is increased there is less energy for the minerals and enzymes to connect and reactions happen more slowly.

Distinct fluids have different ideal pH readings. Normally blood is slightly alkaline with a reading between 7.35 and 7.45 pH. The acid/alkaline balance in the blood must be maintained on a daily basis. Calcium that is stored in the bone is used to keep the blood pH in balance. The pH of the urine should not get too alkaline, but should stay somewhat acid. The saliva pH must not be too acid. Optimal first morning readings after fasting all night for saliva is 6.4 to 6.8 pH, and for urine 6.0 to 6.4 pH. The urine pH reading should be lower than saliva pH in the morning since the urine is dumping residues from nighttime fasting. However, when the urine pH is under 6.0 for a long period of time the body begins to age more quickly, and enzymes needed to rebuild cells are inactivated. As the urine pH gets above 6.4, it shows that the metabolism is moving more slowly, and problems such as constipation may be occurring.

Each body system has its own preferred pH level that shifts during the day. Overall, the body's internal chemical environment normally changes from a weak acid to a weak base within a 24-hour period, usually more acid in the morning and more base in the evening. The slightly acid time period in the early morning is optimal for the activity of the nerves, hormones and neurotransmitters. During the morning, the acid wastes are dissolved and eliminated in the urine. During the day, the body buffers the pH of the food and beverages consumed by releasing electrolytes, and then the pH level goes up. This process allows the kidneys to keep the elimination process balanced. When the pH level gets too high it indicates that the body is buffering with ammonia to compensate for a bio-chemical system that is too acid. Generally, when urine pH level stays below 6.0 for an extended period of time, it is an indication that the body's fluids elsewhere are too acid, and it is working overtime to get rid of the excess acids. When the urine pH is too acid, the body releases many electrolytes to keep the pH level normal and maintain life.

There are two easy and convenient tests that give an accurate indication of the pH of your internal environment. They are performed with the use of pH litmus paper that measures the pH level of the saliva and urine. The most commonly used pH papers register pH values from a moderately strong acid pH of 5.5 to a mildly alkaline pH of 8.0. The thin strip of orange-yellow paper turns color when it comes into contact with moist, or wet, acid or alkaline substances. Matching the color of the exposed litmus paper to the color on the color guide, and recording the numerical value indicated determine the pH value.

The pH of your saliva moves from high to low according to what you eat during the day, and how your body metabolizes your food. To test for saliva pH, use a strip of pH test paper two inches long and create a pool of saliva on your tongue. While holding one end of the test paper, dip the other end into the saliva being careful not to touch your lips to the paper. After dipping in the saliva, immediately pull it out and read the level according to the chart. It is important to read the paper immediately because as the paper sits in the open air the color can change, especially if it is an alkaline reading. Take a reading upon first rising in the morning. Ideally, the saliva pH reading should be between 6.4 and 6.8. If it is lower than 6.4 pH, it indicates that acid wastes are in your saliva in the morning. Test it again during the day about two hours after eating to see if the saliva pH is stable during the day. Keep a record to see the average saliva pH in the morning and during the day. If the pH value varies considerably during the day, it indicates a need to make dietary changes. It will be necessary to change the type of foods being consumed. It is also very important to get the proper amounts of vitamins and minerals to support the body chemistry.

Salvia pH readings reflect the health of the lymph system, the upper digestive system including the stomach, pancreas and liver, and the state of the sympathetic and parasympathetic nervous system. The saliva contains an enzyme that comes directly from the liver. So the saliva pH is a good indicator of the strength of the liver. The saliva pH reveals the level of energy coming into the body. Urine pH indicates the overall function of cell metabolism, showing the level of metabolic wastes being removed. When the urine and saliva pH are both acid, the whole system moves too rapidly, and more energy is used to break down tissue than to rebuild tissue. On the reverse side, when the body is too alkaline the system moves more slowly.

Urine testing is best done upon first rising in the morning. Since the body is removing wastes overnight the body will tend to be more acid in the morning. During the day the ideal urine pH is 6.4, but first thing in the morning it can range from 6.0 to 6.4 pH. Urine testing is best done by testing the urine in mid-stream, using either a cup to catch the urine or by using a longer strip of pH paper.

The urine pH shows the level of acidity of the cell metabolism. The pH of urine may range from 4.5 to 8.0 pH. The kidneys maintain normal pH balance primarily by retaining sodium and secreting hydrogen and ammonium ions. Urine becomes increasingly acid as the amount of sodium and excess acid retained by the body increases. Alkaline urine is normally excreted when there is an excess of base or alkaline substances in the body. Secretion of an acid or alkaline urine by the kidneys is one of the most important mechanisms the body uses to maintain a constant body pH.

A highly acid urine pH occurs in uncontrolled diabetes, diarrhea, dehydration, and respiratory diseases in which carbon dioxide retention occurs. Highly alkaline urine occurs in urinary tract obstruction, kidney weakness, and respiratory diseases that involve hyperventilation. Most of the bacteria responsible for urinary tract infections make the urine more alkaline because the bacteria split the urea into ammonia and other alkaline waste products. The formation of kidney stones is related to the urine pH. Patients being treated for certain types of kidney stones are frequently given diets or medications to change the pH of the urine so that kidney stones will decrease. Calcium phosphate, calcium carbonate, and magnesium phosphate stones develop in alkaline urine. Therefore, in this case, the urine should be kept acid. Uric acid, cystine, and calcium oxalate stones form in acid urine, and in this situation the urine should be kept alkaline or less acid than normal.

What exactly do low pH numbers mean? When the pH of the urine or saliva continues to be less than 6.0, the state of health is varies between mildly poor to very poor. Anxiety or chronic stress could also be affecting the physiology. If mental or emotional factors are not the cause, improving diet, detoxification and gentle exercise will move the values up to the correct range. When the saliva pH is at least 6.2 it is within the healing range, which indicates that the body has the ability to come back into balance more easily with simple changes in diet. Keeping a diet diary along with your saliva and urine pH readings will show what foods are causing your body to be too acid.

Maintaining a balanced pH is important. The pH level has a strong effect on the chemistry of our bodily fluids, either creating health or disease. Our metabolism functions more effectively with a balanced pH. Most of the regulatory processes including digestion, circulation, and breathing are altered to maintain the best pH possible. The longer the pH is out of balance the worse the metabolism functions. Toxins will build-up more quickly and more damage will occur to our cells. The body will use acid-neutralizing minerals, such as calcium that is stored in the bones, to maintain a healthy balance. This is why as we get older we have a greater tendency toward osteoporosis.

"Acidosis," is the term used to describe an imbalanced acid condition of all our body fluids. Acidosis is a condition that occurs when too many hydrogen ions are measured in body fluids. Virtually all functions of the body are sensitive to the pH levels of their fluids. If the pH deviates too far to the acid side, cells become poisoned in their own toxic acid wastes and die. Acidosis seriously obstructs the activities of enzymes involved in the digestive system, the nervous system and the energy operations of the body. Acidosis is caused by oxidative stress that builds up, eventually causing an increase in hydrogen ions. Acidosis also comes from weakened oxygen metabolism in the cells and tissues. An acid pH, if left unchecked, will interrupt all cellular activities and functions, including the regularity of your heart rate and the brain function required to remember simple things. When cells are blocked by toxins or by a lack of cell flexibility, oxygen is unable to penetrate into the individual cell. The cell begins to starve. This in turn causes pain, fatigue, and many of the other symptoms related to fibromyalgia.

Some of the common symptoms of being too acid are tiredness, catching colds easily, pain in the muscles and connective tissues, which produce headaches, stomachaches and tightness in the chest. When the acid condition continues over a long period of time, excess acid substances will be deposited in weakened areas of the body, so that the blood will able to be maintained in it's essential alkaline level. The cells around these weakened areas will either die, or try to adapt to this acid environment. Since these cells are too acid, when these cells try to adapt, they can become malignant abnormal cells, creating cancer and other chronic disorders in the body.

Chronic disorders are non-contagious health conditions that we develop slowly, most often, as we get older. In addition to fibromyalgia, some other examples of chronic disorders are heart disease, high blood pressure, diabetes, arthritis, gout, asthma, hay fever, allergies, headaches, psoriasis, and obesity. The most common causes of these chronic disorders are the accumulation of acids in our body, poor blood circulation and poor cell activity.

The pharmaceutical companies continue to do research on medications to cure every type of chronic disorder. Chronic disorders are often caused by an acid / alkaline imbalance, so unless the treatment actually balances the cellular fluids, the 'cure' at best will be only temporary. None of these drugs reduce the acidity in the body. As a matter of a fact, most drugs make the body more acid. When the body extracts alkaline minerals from its cells to neutralize the acid, it causes the cells to become acid, and thus diseased. To maintain health the majority of our diet must consist of alkaline foods.

What makes a food more alkaline is the presence of organic minerals. When minerals are inherently in the food, then that food is alkaline. Foods do not become alkaline by enriching them with inorganic minerals. The Standard American Diet is high in protein, high in carbohydrate, high in fat and very little, if not completely inadequate, in the amount of fruits and vegetables. The most commonly eaten foods are acid forming foods and will keep the body chemistry more acid. Changing the diet is the best approach to maintain appropriate pH levels throughout the body. When food is metabolized and broken down, it creates either acid or alkaline pH levels in the tissues. Certain foods are acid forming in nature, whereas others are known to be alkaline-forming.

Most high protein foods, such as meat, fish, poultry and eggs, nearly all carbohydrates, including grains, breads, pastas, and fats are acid-forming. Most fruits and vegetables are alkaline forming. Although citrus fruits, such as oranges and grapefruit, contain organic acids and may have an acid taste, they are not acid forming when metabolized, and can actually make the tissues more alkaline.

The National Cancer Institute recommends that all Americans get at least 5 servings per day of fruits and vegetables. Yet, most Americans do not get half that amount. To prevent cancer we need 10 to 12 servings of fruits and vegetables per day. Why is this? Fruits and vegetables are alkalizing to the system creating more oxygen in the cells. Cancer cannot live in an oxygenated environment. Daily amounts of fruits and vegetables are a dietary change that is absolutely necessary to maintain health.

By consuming a diet that is 70-80% alkaline and 20-30% acid, we can stay healthy. The more alkaline foods we daily the better we will feel. If we become too alkaline by eating a majority of alkaline foods, we will lose our appetite and automatically want to fast, during which time the normal acid metabolic by-products will return the body' s pH level back to normal.

There are many choices that can assist, on a short or long-term basis to make the cells more alkaline. One of the fastest ways to change from an acid state to a more neutral state is to make an alkaline broth. To make this broth, combine four different alkaline vegetables, such as onions, kelp, yams, parsnips, garlic, broccoli, and/or kale and simmer slowly in water. After the vegetables have cooked and become soft, remove the vegetables and drink the broth. Drink at least one cup of broth per day, up to three cups for a highly acid state. This broth has all the alkalizing minerals that will change the pH of the cells toward the alkaline side.

Make sure that your choice of drinks, including water, is in the neutral pH range. Soda pop is very acid with a pH between 2.0 and 3.0 pH. Coffee is also acid, as is black tea. However, green tea is an alkalizing drink, and is a good choice to bring your cells back to a more neutral pH. Most types of water, with minerals still in them, are in the neutral pH range, from 6.5 to 7.5 pH. If you filter your water, make sure that the pH is still in the healthy range, or it will cause more stress on your cells.

There are various charts of acid and alkaline foods. Some foods begin as acids, yet when they are metabolized they actually create an alkaline reaction.

Some examples of the foods that create an alkaline reaction but initially have an acid reaction are oranges, lemons, and apple cider vinegar. When adding sugar to any food it makes it more acid. Also, the more processed the food, the more acid it will be, due to the preservatives in the food. The following list shows foods that tend to create acid and alkaline conditions.

Acid Creating Foods

Fruits:
    cranberry
    blueberry
    dried fruits

Nuts and Grains:
    oats
    barley
    rice
    wheat
    white bread
    peanuts
    walnuts
    processed soybeans

Other:
    sugar
    chocolate
    honey
    aspirin
    white vinegar

Vegetables:
    corn, processed

Meats and Dairy Products:
    beef
    veal
    turkey
    chicken
    ham
    haddock
    milk and cheese
    yogurt
    ice cream
    butter

Drinks:
    coffee
    beer
    black tea
    soft drinks

Alkaline Creating Foods

Fruits:

    apricots
    melons
    raspberries
    tart cherries
    mangos
    bananas
    grapes
    grapefruit
    orange
    lemon
    lime
    pineapples
    pears
    apples
    peaches
    nectarines
    watermelon
    strawberries
    tangerines
    plums

Nuts and Grains:

    almonds
    alfalfa sprouts
    beans
    molasses
    millet
    quinoa
    green soybeans

Vegetables:

    collard greens
    sweet potatoes
    mushrooms
    corn on the cob
    cabbage
    broccoli
    Brussels sprouts
    onions
    parsnips
    beets
    dark leafy greens
    cauliflower
    carrots
    tomatoes
    kelp
    kale
    celery
    green peppers
    parsley
    spinach
    peas
    green beans

Drinks:

    green tea

Other:

    apple cider vinegar

Many reports exist explaining the benefits of using apple cider vinegar to improve health. This is because of its alkaline producing properties. The apple cider vinegar has to be pure, or the taste will be offensive. Green tea contains many antioxidants and phytochemicals, along with minerals that make it an alkaline drink. Green tea has many benefits and even though it contains some caffeine, is a much better choice of drink than coffee or soft drinks.

Bio-Chemical Testing for Acidosis

Saliva and urine are the most convenient extra-cellular fluids that can be used to measure the biological "terrain" which shows the overall health level. This terrain is constantly shifting depending on the demands that are placed on it. Every thought, feeling, and physical experience, including every stress and every bite of food eaten by the body affects the bio-chemical systems. A variety of non-invasive saliva and urine tests measure the various chemical reactions that monitor changes in health.

One way of determining your tendency toward problems relating to imbalances in pH readings is to keep a record of your daily pH readings on the following chart. The two intersecting lines come together at a pH of 6.4, with the urine pH going vertically from 5.0 at the bottom of the chart to 8.0 at the top of the chart. The saliva pH is the horizontal line beginning at 5.0 pH on the left side and going to 8.0 pH on the right edge. By plotting your different pH readings daily, you can see which area most of your readings are located. The more often your readings are within the triangle in the middle of the chart, the better your potential health level. The triangle contains the area of healthy pH levels. The triangle area represents the urine pH readings between 6.0 and 6.4, and the saliva pH readings between 6.4 and 6.8.

Patterns of Stress

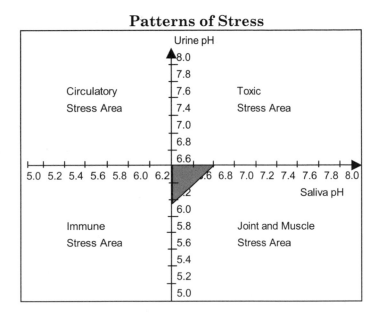

This chart shows the four imbalances that create certain types of condition patterns. When the urine and saliva pH both are too high, there is a tendency to toxic conditions in the metabolism. When the urine pH is low and the saliva pH is high, there is a tendency toward joint and muscle stress or pain from congestion in these tissues. When the urine pH is high and the saliva pH is low, it can lead to stress in the circulatory system. Finally, when both the urine and saliva pH are low consistently, it leads to immune stress, where oxidative stress is causing the body to age more quickly. The ideal region is within the triangle where the ideal urine and saliva ranges are located.

When both the urine and saliva pH are too high for a period of time, above 6.4 pH for urine, and above 6.8 pH for saliva, then the body goes into a toxic stress state. When this occurs the system is overloaded, producing constipation and congestion. Symptoms of intestinal gas, body odors, bad breath, and a distended abdomen occur. Other symptoms related to this toxic stress state are sinus and upper respiratory congestion, skin discoloration, disk deterioration along the spine, and increased tooth decay. Alkaline pH readings indicate that the metabolism has slowed down, and can be caused by liver or kidney weakness.

When the saliva pH is above 6.8 and the urine is lower than 6.0 then the body goes into a state of joint and muscle stress. The digestive system is out of balance since the upper digestive system is moving slower than the lower digestive system, creating abdominal gas and bloating. This combination creates congestion and accumulation of toxins, generating knots and lumps in the soft tissues. Energy is being lost in the system. Fibromyalgia pain in the tender points comes from these toxins that have accumulated in the muscle tissues.

When the saliva pH is low, below 6.4, and the urine pH measures above 6.4, then there is a tendency toward slow circulation, with a movement toward having a stroke or heart attack. Also in this pattern there is digestive stress since in this case the upper digestive system is moving quickly and the colon area is shifting toward a slow state. Excess wastes that are created when the body is too acid are unable to move out of the system. This is what causes the circulation problems, since the toxins created cannot be released as necessary.

When the saliva pH stays lower than 6.4 and the urine pH is lower than 6.0 for a period of time, then the immune system is affected. This acid state occurs because the digestive system is moving too fast and nutrients cannot get into the cells. There will be a tendency toward fungal infections, leg cramping and joint aching. The calcium will be drawn out of the bones to balance this acid state, so osteoporosis occurs when the body stays in this pattern. When the urine and saliva measurements test regularly with lowered pH readings, less oxygen is in the cells. This lack of oxygen in the tissues increases anaerobic bacteria and fungal growth in the body. This immune system stress will cause shortness of breath, since the lungs will be drawn upon for mineral energy. Chronic diarrhea and other malabsorption problems will be seen, such as colitis and Crohn's disease. Also, anemia comes from prolonged acid conditions, and even supplementing vitamin B-12 and iron will not help unless pH levels are improved.

The biochemical research study results revealed that 54% of the fibromyalgia participants had saliva and urine pH results in the immune stress area, and 30% of the pH readings were in the joint and muscle stress area. Only 6% percent of the fibromyalgia group had readings in the circulatory stress area, and only 2% in the toxic stress area. Just 8% of the combined saliva and urine pH readings for the fibromyalgia group were in the ideal triangular shaped area.

Saliva pH Challenge Test

The Saliva pH Challenge Test is a simple saliva test that helps monitor the mineral reserves in the metabolism, and shows how the nervous system reacts to stress. Minerals are needed along with enzymes for every cell activity. In this test, reactions that come from adequate mineral reserves are monitored after drinking an acid lemon juice and water combination. The reactions are measured every minute for five minutes. These pH readings, taken every minute, show the sympathetic nervous system's stress response. This test also shows if there are enough minerals in the tissues to react appropriately to stress.

The Saliva pH Challenge Test plots the following information on the chart:

1. the baseline saliva pH
2. the initial pH reaction to drinking a small amount of lemon juice and water, and
3. the minute-by-minute pH level reactions to the acid lemon juice.

The following chart shows the ideal minute-by-minute response to the Saliva pH Challenge Test:

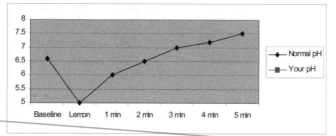

When the results of each pH test are graphed, the difference in the readings from the ideal points indicate the degree of sympathetic nervous system stress, the potential adrenal stress, and the amount of minerals ready to respond to stress.[12] By looking at the graph of the pH readings over time, the following can be determined:

1. Are there enough minerals, specifically magnesium and potassium, to deal with daily stresses?
2. Is the body responding too quickly or slowly to stress?
3. Are additional minerals needed to improve the stress response?

In the research study, this graph was charted for each participant. Since, many people do not have ideal test results, but also do not have fibromyalgia, the control group readings were compared to the readings for the fibromyalgia group. The following table shows the various averages for the different saliva tests. The baseline saliva pH levels ideally should be in the 6.4 to 6.8 pH range. The saliva pH-1 reading is the part of the Saliva pH Acid Challenge test where the reaction to the lemon juice was recorded 1-minute after drinking it. The Saliva pH-1 stands for the 1-minute reading, and the Saliva pH-5 is the 5-minute reading.

Average Results	Fibromyalgia	Control	Ideal
Baseline Saliva pH	6.17	6.35	6.60
Saliva pH-1	6.42	6.76	6.40
Saliva pH-5	6.24	6.64	7.40

The above chart shows that the average baseline saliva pH is lower in people who have been diagnosed with fibromyalgia. This reading was done during the daytime hours at least one hour after eating, so the affect of food was minimal. The saliva pH-5 level shows the level of available minerals, such as potassium and magnesium, which were able to create an alkaline reaction to the lemon juice. The ideal alkaline reading is the normal reaction when enough minerals are on hand. When the saliva pH-5 is less than 7.0 then more minerals, especially magnesium and potassium, are needed. The saliva pH-5 average was much lower in the fibromyalgia group, showing that the existing mineral supply was so low that the liver could not create a normal alkaline reaction. The saliva pH-1 average reading was higher in the control group and will be explained further in the following chart.

Percentage of Low Readings	Fibromyalgia	Control
Baseline Saliva pH <6.2	42%	24%
Saliva pH-1 <5.6	32%	20%
Saliva pH-1 >6.8	54%	50%
Saliva pH-5 <6.2	36%	8%

This chart shows the percentage of saliva readings that were out of balance when the baseline saliva pH was less than 6.2, when saliva pH-1 was too high or too low, and when the final reading for saliva pH-5 was less than 6.2. From this chart you can see that 42% of the fibromyalgia group has lower baseline saliva pH readings, compared to only 24% of people in the control group.

The next two lines in the chart show the low saliva pH-1 readings and the high saliva pH-1 readings. When the saliva pH does not respond quickly to the lemon juice the 1-minute reading will be low. The readings below 5.6 pH indicate an inability for the nervous system to react to stress. The fibromyalgia group had 32% with this weak nervous system response, compared to 20% in the control group.

When the saliva pH-1 reading is above 6.8, it indicates a quick sympathetic nervous system response. In this case, the nervous system responded quickly to the stress from the acid lemon juice and used up minerals, or ammonia, to create this increased reaction. One-half of the people in the control group had this quick nervous system response compared to 54% in the fibromyalgia group.

The saliva pH-5 reading should be higher than the initial baseline pH. This reading shows the 5-minute response to the lemon juice. Ideally, the lemon juice will create an alkaline reaction in the liver, and therefore in the saliva. When there is not an alkaline reaction, then the body is very low on available minerals and cannot respond to stress adequately. The chart shows that 36% of the fibromyalgia participants had a very low alkaline reaction, compared to only 8% in the control group.

This Saliva pH Challenge Test shows many types of potential mineral depletion risk factors and responses to stress. One response to stress is when the baseline pH and all of the following pH readings at 1-minute intervals, are below 5.5 on the pH measurement. This indicates that there is a lack of response in the nervous system, and presents the possibility of serious organ weakness. In this case, there is such a lack of energy that the body is not able to respond to stress efficiently. The research study revealed that many individuals who were taking four or more types of prescription drugs, or who were heavy users of antacids, had this lack of response. This shows that slowing the digestion in the stomach with antacids causes a lowered pH and weakening of the digestive response. Synthetic prescription drugs are known to increase free radicals in the body and to cause more acidity in the metabolism.

Calcium Level Test

Calcium is the most abundant mineral found in the body, located mostly in the bones and teeth. Pure calcium is the most alkaline mineral. When calcium supplements are taken, they help to sustain the acid and alkaline balance. Calcium helps to maintain healthy bones and teeth, improve muscle response including the contraction of the heart muscle, improve nerve impulse contraction, release neurotransmitters, activate cell enzymes, and regulate blood calcium levels by borrowing from the bone when necessary.

The Calcium Level test mixes a reagent of oxalic acid, ammonium oxalate and glacial acetic acid with equal amounts of urine. Then the solution is observed for turbidity, or cloudiness.[13] The reagent contains oxalate chemicals buffered so that calcium will almost immediately show up as a faint white haze. A clear solution indicates low calcium. A moderate cloudy solution indicates normal calcium levels, and a milky or thick cloudy solution indicates excess calcium, or hypercalcaemia.

In the research study, the Calcium test results showed that people diagnosed with fibromyalgia had considerably less available calcium than people in the control group. 70% of the participants diagnosed with fibromyalgia had low calcium reserves, compared to only 24% in the control group. Calcium is the mineral that balances the pH reserves and helps to maintain a steady biochemistry. It is the most important mineral to get in your diet and absorb from your supplements.

---

[12] Yanick, Paul, and Jaffe Russell, *"Clinical Chemistry and Nutrition: A Physician's Desk Reference."* Lake Ariel, PA: T&H Publishing

[13] Goske C., *"Use of Random Urine Samples to Estimate Total Urinary Calcium and Phosphate Excretion."* Arch. Int. Med. 151(8):1587-1588, Aug. 1991.

13

Overall Research Test Results

The interacting physical systems that can be monitored by measuring biological terrain are the nervous system, endocrine system, digestive system, and lymphatic system. By looking at the urine and saliva pH levels, the mineral levels, the oxidation levels, and the adrenal stress levels, the terrain of the whole system can be measured. In addition to using the first morning's urine and saliva pH readings to determine potential acidosis, the other tests show cause and effect of oxidative stress and acid conditions. Each specific test, other than urine pH, has been discussed already. Now, we will look at the effects of urine pH levels, and combine those results with the other tests to see the collective results common to people diagnosed with fibromyalgia.

The first morning urine pH levels should be between 6.0 and 6.4. In this research project the average first morning urine pH for people in the fibromyalgia group was 5.56 pH, compared to 5.90 pH in the control group. Also, there were 74% of the people in the fibromyalgia group with a pH reading below 6.0, compared to only 24% in the control group. This data shows that there is a greater tendency toward lower urine pH in people who have the symptoms of fibromyalgia. This acid condition in the metabolism definitely could be a factor in the cause of the constant pain. Remember that the urine pH level reveals how well the cell metabolism is functioning and the quantity of metabolic wastes being removed. When metabolic acids build up in the muscles, pain is the most common consequence. The following graph shows the saliva and urine pH levels for the fibromyalgia group and the control group, compared to the ideal readings. You can see that the average pH level of the participants with fibromyalgia is lower than the control group and the ideal readings.

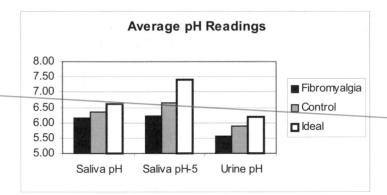

When other tests are combined with the urine pH reading it demonstrates how the levels of acidity are affecting the body. The urine pH value is a good overall view of metabolic health, and the tendency toward acidosis. If calcium is low, there is a greater tendency toward acidity. When calcium and the urine pH is low, there is a greater tendency toward stress or metabolic acidosis. This can come from eating too much protein in the diet, or it can be a factor of the adrenal response. The actual urine pH readings combined with the saliva pH readings after an acid stress test, are other good indicators of the tendency toward acidosis. When all tests are looked at in combination they can indicate if there is truly an acidosis condition that may be creating the pain of fibromyalgia.

The following table shows by percentage how often imbalances occurred when combining the results low urine pH with other tests. These comparisons look at the different extremes in the various tests. In this chart, the higher percentage is seen most often in the fibromyalgia group indicating that imbalances are occurring more often in that group.

Percentage of Low Readings	Fibromyalgia	Control
Urine pH <6.0	74%	24%
Saliva pH<6.2 + Urine pH<6	34%	16%
Saliva pH-1<5.6 + Urine pH<6	30%	12%
Saliva pH-5>6.2 + Urine pH<6	30%	4%
Adrenal<13 + Urine pH<6	20%	6%
Adrenal>25 + Urine pH<6	24%	14%
Calcium=0 + Urine pH<6	60%	12%

The following graph compares the saliva readings when the urine reading is also low. When both of the urine and saliva readings are low, there is more of a tendency toward acidosis. This indicates that the body is breaking down faster than it is rebuilding. This graph is showing that the Fibromyalgia group (34%) has a greater tendency toward lower baseline pH when the urine pH is also low, than the control group (16%). At the 1-minute reading when the saliva pH measured less than 5.6, and the urine pH was less than 6.0, the fibromyalgia group had 30% in this range compared to 12% in the control group. The results for the 5-minute reading for saliva pH under 6.2, and urine pH below 6.0, again showed that the fibromyalgia group was noticeably more out of balanced than the control group, by a difference of 26%. All these numbers indicate that when the urine pH is low, the body shows a greater sympathetic nervous system imbalance, with symptoms of lower nerve response, which create hypersensitivity to pain.

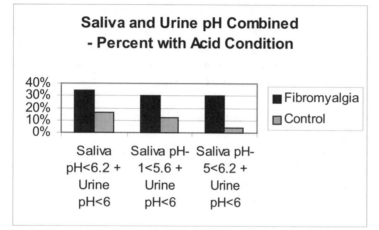

The following graph shows the percentage of participants with low pH urine reading along with adrenal stress, adrenal fatigue, and low calcium levels. Calcium levels have a direct correlation to the acid/alkaline balance in the body. When calcium is lacking in the urine, the system will tend to become more acid. In this study, 60% of the Fibromyalgia group, as compared to 12% of the control group, was low in calcium along with having a lowered urine pH reading. This graph also shows that the fibromyalgia group had more adrenal weakness, when the urine pH was also below normal, than the control group. This continued weakness in the adrenals causes a lack of energy in the tissues, leading to the painful symptoms of fibromyalgia. To counteract lowered calcium, and the lack of other minerals as seen by the imbalances in the

Adrenal Stress test and the Saliva pH Challenge test, it is necessary to get the metabolism in balance so that these minerals are absorbed effectively. This can be done with the use of enzymes and essential fatty acids.

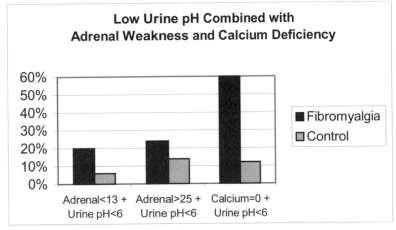

The findings of this bio-chemical study show a considerable difference between the results of people who have been diagnosed with fibromyalgia and those in the control group. Acidosis states are definitely more common in the fibromyalgia group along with lowered mineral reserves. Also, adrenal stress is more common in fibromyalgia patients, which indicates that there is a continued stress response within the body. There is also a lack of antioxidants and a greater amount of free radicals in the fibromyalgia group. All of these tests combined show that fibromyalgia symptoms can be caused by a weakened metabolism affecting the nervous system and circulatory system. By acquiring good levels of calcium, magnesium, potassium, and organic sodium in the system, and by improving digestion, stress will have less effect on the body. This will reduce the painful symptoms of fibromyalgia.

∞14∞

Part III

Designing Your Own Program
To Reverse Fibromyalgia Symptoms

Many factors will influence the length of time it will take for you to reverse your fibromyalgia symptoms. By learning how to incorporate various aspects of this program into your daily lifestyle, you will have the best likelihood to create the health you desire. A variety of causes of fibromyalgia symptoms, and the effects of environmental stresses have been discussed already. Something as simple as taking in more water can make a huge difference. Many people have realized a major change just by changing from carbonated drinks to regular water. Learning how to get the proper rest and exercise has helped with sleep patterns and fatigue.

The level of vitality in your body is dependent on the level of cell acidity, the amount of accumulated toxins, and the degree of degeneration of your body tissues. Yet, mental factors such as anxiety level and thought processes also affect your health. Do you talk to yourself in a positive manner, or do you have a tendency to put yourself down? What level of worry do you hold inside your body on a daily basis? The amount of self-discipline, willingness and determination you possess are factors that will greatly influence your ability in making in lifestyle changes. The clients that were

totally determined to feel better made the changes
necessary to become healthier. Understanding how true
healing occurs, and being determined to incorporate
some required changes to create healing, will enable the
healing process to transpire. There is a saying "The
definition of insanity is expecting things to change when
you haven't." The patterns of our health come on from
habits in our lives. Changing lifestyle, dietary,
emotional, and mental habits will transform our healing
ability. Generally it takes one year of healing for every
four years of living a toxic lifestyle, or one month for
every four months. Everyone is different, so
improvements are dependent on the strength of the
whole body, including the mental and emotional
stability.

Much of the research on fibromyalgia states that,
in part, the symptoms are caused by fibrous reactions to
chemical imbalances in the body, which may in turn, be
partly caused by dietary imbalances. Many people with
fibromyalgia have discovered that changing their diet
has made quite a difference to their symptoms. These
dietary changes are necessary because the current diet
has a harmful effect on the tissues, particularly the
muscles, which over time have become fibrous, or
hardened, and less able to function properly.
Fibromyalgia patients have the ability to reduce pain by
providing the body with the nutrients it needs to
function well, and to replace the nutrients that are
depleted on a daily basis. As we have previously
discussed, it is recommended to avoid acid forming foods
like sugary and processed foods, caffeine and carbonated
drinks

The participants in the study used many
different types of nutritional supplements to relieve the
symptoms of fibromyalgia. The most common type of

supplements used were multiple vitamin and mineral supplements, and calcium, both at 28%. Vitamin C was next at 24%. Magnesium and B complex were the other two most common nutritional supplements used. All of these supplements will be discussed along with others that are also necessary.

Energy is created from food by breaking it down into individual atoms so the nutrients can be passed into individual cells. This takes place within the mitochondria, the structures within cells that provide the energy required by most of the chemical reactions vital to normal health. Over 80 nutrients are needed for proper metabolism and energy production. If sufficient amounts are not provided, the metabolism will be impaired and degenerative disease will occur more often.

Addressing and reversing the problem of nutrient deficiencies enhance the healing process. Pain, stress, anxiety, and depression use up the minerals that the body must have for proper functioning. The brain must constantly be replenished with needed nutrients. Supplying the proper type of nutrients, in the correct proportions, will have a positive effect on pain, anxiety and depression that accompany fibromyalgia.

❧15❧

Antioxidants and Free Radicals

Decreasing our exposure to risk factors that create free radicals is just the beginning of staying healthy. It is impossible to eliminate all free radicals without the support of antioxidants. There must be enough antioxidants available to handle all of the free radicals produced, or oxidative stress will create degenerative diseases. Free radicals inflict some damage on our cells, even when we have adequate antioxidants. However, the body does have a great ability to heal itself with the proper nutrients.

When there is a lot of stress or acidity in the system, free radicals will thrive. Excess free radical activity comes from an impaired metabolism or an immune system response to environmental toxins or allergens. Free radicals are highly reactive chemical ions. They cause microscopic tissue damage to body proteins producing hardening in the soft tissues. As a highly reactive chemical agent, a free radical will combine with other ions that are in the vicinity. This coming together of ions is called oxidation and often sets off a chain reaction that can lead to very negative results. When free radicals are made in the body, the body tissues become stressed and cause abnormal cells. If not counteracted, chronic diseases, such as cancer or fibromyalgia, develop depending on the areas of weakness in the body. Increasing dietary antioxidants, along with increasing the amount of enzymes and minerals, will offset free radical damage in the cells

The body has the ability to make some of its own antioxidants. Two of them are called superoxide dismutase (SOD) and catalase. However, the body is not able to produce enough of these antioxidants on its own to neutralize all of the free radicals present. Adequate amounts of antioxidants need to be supplied daily through our food and the use of supplements. The most common antioxidants are vtamins A, C and E.

Vitamin C is water-soluble and the most effective antioxidant for the health of the blood. Vitamin C is essential for the health of the connective tissue, and the support of bones, blood vessels, joints, organs, muscles, eyes, teeth and skin. Vitamin C helps with antibody production and white blood cell activity. It can help reduce cholesterol and protects your heart. Since it is water-soluble it protects the watery tissues of your body including your sinuses. Vitamin C also helps to manufacture neurotransmitters like serotonin and dopamine, protects the gall bladder from gallstones, and improves the transport of iron into cells.

Vitamin E is a fat-soluble vitamin and the most effective antioxidant for the health of the cell wall. Vitamin E is found in four major tocopherols compounds called alpha-tocopherols, beta-tocopherols, gamma-tocopherols, and delta tochopherols. The most common form of Vitamin E in supplements is alpha-tocopherol. All of the tocopherols are found in whole vegetables, and work together to support the immune and circulatory systems. Vitamin E destroys free radicals, helps to heal the skin, fights disease and helps reduce heart problems. Also, vitamin E is beneficial in reversing calcium build-up in the soft tissue and easing stiffness in the connective tissue. When consumed together, Vitamin C improves the effectiveness of vitamin E, and may block some of the harmful effects of a high fat meal

Vitamin A is another fat-soluble nutrient stored in the liver. It comes into the body from beta-carotene, one of the twenty-two carotenoids found in fruits and vegetables. Vitamin A is needed for the health of the immune system, and helps with reproduction of cells in the respiratory and digestive tract. It is also necessary for good night vision, and helps to prevent dry eyes. This is why our mothers told us to eat carrots. The orange color in the carrot is full of carotenoids and therefore helps with many aspects of our vision. By combining vitamin A with all the other antioxidant vitamins the metabolic process will be more efficient, excess free radicals will be decreased, energy levels will improve and pain will subside. There must always be an abundant supply of antioxidants within every cell and tissue to protect the body against free radicals.

In addition to these vitamins, there are thousands of other antioxidants obtained from foods, primarily fruits and vegetables. **Phytochemicals**, or plant chemicals that have the strongest antioxidant properties, are found in fruits and vegetables. The various colors reveal the benefit of the fruits and vegetables. Deeper colors indicate a greater amount of phytochemicals. Red foods help strengthen the blood. Green foods have the whole vitamin E compound and benefit the circulatory system. Orange colored foods have many antioxidants including vitamins A and C. There are more than one thousand types of phytochemicals. An apple has more than 300 different phytochemicals that help to improve our health when we eat the apple. The greater the variety of phytochemicals available to the body, the better chance for free radicals to be reduced.

There is no way all of the phytochemicals can be broken down effectively into separate supplements. It is best to get them from the daily diet or whole food supplements. Alpha lipoic acid, mixed carotenoids, Coenzyme Q10, indoles, N-acetyl-N cysteine, lutein, and bioflavonoids are examples of identified phytochemicals available in whole foods to help us in the battle against free radicals. Sulfurophane is a phytochemical found in broccoli that helps to shrink cancerous tumors. But it does not work effectively unless combined with all of the other phytochemicals in the broccoli. Not only do these phytochemicals and antioxidants work in synergy with one another, but also they work against different types of free radicals.

How many antioxidants do you need? Vitamins A, C and E are more easily metabolized and absorbed into the system when taken grouped together, than when taken separately. The commonly recommended dosages of vitamin A is 5000 I.U., vitamin C is 500 mg, and vitamin E is 400 I.U. per day. Eating the standard American diet, which includes many saturated fats from meats, or hydrogenated oils from processed foods, more free radicals will be created, and there will be a need for additional antioxidants. These fats do not break down in the system. Excessive cholesterol is created to protect the arteries from the free radicals that are produced from eating these fats. Individuals need to take higher doses of antioxidants with these fatty meals, so that these effects are can be eliminated. Also, if you have tendency to sinus congestion, or have a susceptibility to colds and other viruses, then you will need additional antioxidants.

Antioxidants by themselves are not the complete answer. They work more efficiently with adequate amounts of minerals, including trace minerals such as copper, zinc, manganese, and selenium. Also, there must be adequate amounts of cofactors such as folic acid and vitamins B1, B2, B6, and B12. These nutrients are essential in the enzymatic reactions of the antioxidants. If these minerals and B complex vitamins are not present in adequate amounts, even when antioxidants are present, oxidative stress will still occur.

Juice Plus+

For many years, one of the most commonly recommended supplements that I have used for fibromyalgia clients is called Juice Plus+. Juice Plus+ is a concentrated fruit and vegetable supplement that contains digestive enzymes and other nutrients that are highly absorbable in our digestive system. The body is designed to handle whole foods and ideally should get most of its vitamins and minerals from fruits and vegetables. Since Juice Plus+ contains just whole fruits and vegetables, the phytochemical nutrients found in the capsules are beyond measure. Thousands of phytochemicals and minerals are found in fruits and vegetables and are always combined synergistically with other necessary nutrients. The fruits and vegetables found in Juice Plus+ are the most dense and colorful fruits and vegetables. The more variety of color in fruits and vegetables means that there are a greater amount of phytochemicals that are available to act as antioxidants to fight free radicals. We really do not need excess amounts of any one vitamin or mineral. Our bodies can only absorb small amounts of nutrients at one time. When we get too much of any one vitamin, such as vitamin C, it creates an imbalance in other nutrients. The amount of vitamin C found in one orange is just 75 mg. Yet, the orange also contains bioflavonoids and other vitamins and minerals that increase the effectiveness of the natural vitamin C. This is not to that say vitamin and mineral supplements are not necessary for some imbalances, but they are best taken with whole foods where the synergistic effect of all the phytochemicals can work together.

The American Cancer Society recommends that we each eat at least 5 fruits and vegetables daily, and even more to effectively prevent cancer. Yet only 10% of the United States population gets the minimum amounts recommended. The fruits and vegetables should be in a variety of colors to be the most beneficial. Vegetables such as kale, parsley, spinach, broccoli, and beets are very dark in color, which indicates that they are more nutritious. Since Juice Plus+ contains 7 different fruits and 10 different vegetables it gives us the variety of color and nutrients that we need. Juice Plus+ is not made from dehydrated fruits and vegetables. It is made from concentrated fresh juice powders. All the water is removed from the fruit and vegetable juice and the remaining powder is then put into the capsules. It really helps the body maintain a consistent amount of concentrated antioxidants, minerals and enzymes in the digestive system that helps to fight free radicals. Research has been completed on Juice Plus+ that shows that it is very bioavailable, or absorbed easily into the digestive system, thereby improving the level of antioxidants in the blood. It was shown that Juice Plus+ also reduces DNA damage in the body, and improves the function of the immune system.

Other types of whole food antioxidants include some spices we use on our foods, but in higher quantities. We have seen how cayenne pepper has stimulating properties to reduce pain when used in a cream. Another common spice used for fibromyalgia is oregano oil. Oregano is a hot spice with a history of beneficial uses in preserving foods and killing microorganisms in foods. In tablet or capsule form, oregano oil can be taken internally. It works as a potent antioxidant to specifically reduce the growth of toxic bacteria in the intestines. The oxidative stress that is caused by excess candida or other bacterial, viral, or fungal infections is reduced with the use of oregano. Oregano oil is a good choice when the Malabsorption test and/or the Free Radical test have high scores

When taking Juice Plus+, or any other antioxidant food supplement, your body will gradually improve its function. Food supplements need to taken for at least 3 months to recognize their effectiveness. The effects will be cumulative. As the nutrients buildup in your system you will begin to feel the difference good nutrition makes.

✧16✧

Minerals and
Their Specific Role in Cell Activity

The chemical balance of the body depends on the balance of minerals in the system. Each mineral depends on other minerals in a specific ratio to work effectively. Minerals are also known as co-enzymes, working with enzymes to help create energy in the growth and healing of tissue. Minerals specifically help form bones and the blood, keep the nervous system functioning, and regulate the tone of the muscles. There are two types of minerals, macrominerals and trace minerals. The macrominerals are needed in larger amounts than the trace minerals. The macrominerals are calcium, magnesium, potassium, sodium and phosphorus. There are many trace minerals, but the most common are zinc, copper, iron, silicon, manganese, sulfur, chromium, iodine, and selenium. It is possible to create a mineral toxicity from taking too many minerals. However, in order to accumulate too many minerals; they would have to be overly consumed, in inorganic form regularly, for a long period of time.

Calcium is the most abundant mineral found in the body, especially in the bones and teeth, and the rest is in the soft tissues. Calcium is used for muscle contraction and growth, to regulate the nervous system and heart action, to properly clot the blood, to break down fats, and to stabilize protein. Calcium determines the volume and density of each cell, affects the cell's ability to absorb nutrients, and controls the metabolic acids. When there is a calcium deficiency, the muscles cannot effectively absorb any of the minerals they need. Calcium is needed more than any other mineral; yet, it is best absorbed from whole plants instead of by inorganic supplementation. Calcium is found in kelp, almonds, egg yolks, dark leafy green vegetables like kale, spinach, cabbage, and in most dairy products. Sugar in the daily diet depletes calcium, since it increases acidity, which requires the use of more calcium to maintain balance.

In fibromyalgia, calcium is especially needed to balance the acid/alkaline levels and to reduce stress in the muscle and nervous system. The liver needs sufficient amounts of calcium; otherwise, the metabolism of the whole system is affected. There are many types of calcium available on the market. When the pH level is very low, under 5.5, calcium carbonate can be absorbed. At pH levels between 5.5 and 6.2, calcium citrate is absorbed well. When the pH readings are higher than 6.4, calcium lactate is better absorbed. Calcium gluconate is one type of calcium that is absorbed well at all pH levels. Vitamin D is commonly recommended to take with calcium. Actually, it is especially necessary when the pH is too low. The lower the pH the more vitamin D is needed help with calcium absorption. When the pH is on the alkaline side, above 7.0, it is not recommended to supplement vitamin D.

The amount of calcium needed per day is dependent on the form of calcium used, and how well it will be absorbed. Often supplement labels will list the milligrams of calcium and then the amount of elemental calcium. This elemental amount is the actual level of calcium that will be absorbed into the body. When taking over 1000 mg. of calcium to prevent osteoporosis, not all of it will be absorbed, unless is supported with other minerals, such as magnesium, zinc, phosphorus, silica and boron, that it needs to be broken down effectively. Excess calcium that is not absorbed ends up in the tissues, especially in the joints and arteries.

For fibromyalgia, **magnesium** is the most common mineral used to reduce stress in the muscles. Magnesium is the fourth most abundant mineral in the body, and the second most abundant in the muscle tissue. It helps to relax muscles, expand airways, regulate heart rhythm, and is beneficial in nerve formation. Magnesium is needed for over 300 enzyme reactions and is the major mineral required for energy formation. Deficiencies of magnesium can cause swelling of the cell membranes, hardening of the soft tissues, sleep disturbances, and irritability.

Magnesium is one of the most crucial elements for the production of adenosine triphosphate (ATP). The entire energy production system is dependent on magnesium, and even a slight magnesium deficiency can slow down the production of ATP. Oxygen deficiency in the cells can come from lack of magnesium available to the energy cells, or mitochondria. Without the proper amount oxygen and magnesium, lactic acid builds up causing soreness, lung capacity decreases causing shortness of breath, and fatigue increases.

Research shows that many fibromyalgia patients have below-normal levels of magnesium. Low levels of magnesium can also contribute to PMS, headaches, muscle cramping, muscle spasms, heart palpitations and even heart attacks. Many common foods Americans eat do not contain enough magnesium. For example, at least 85 percent of magnesium is removed from bleached and refined flour in breads, pasta and other prepared wheat products. Magnesium is found in whole grains, dark green leafy vegetables, kelp, and many kinds of nuts and legumes.

Soft drinks have a high phosphorus content, which also reduces magnesium levels in the body. Even high calcium supplementation, without adequate magnesium, will deplete the body's level of magnesium. Aluminum toxicity may also play a role in symptoms experienced by people deficient in magnesium, so magnesium supplementation can help block the toxic effects of aluminum. However, the most potent aluminum detoxifier is malic acid. Malic acid is especially effective at decreasing aluminum toxicity in the brain. Clinical tests are proving malic acid to be a great asset in the treatment of fibromyalgia pain especially when in combination with magnesium.

Malic acid in supplementation with magnesium has been shown to improve the amount of oxygen and energy available to the cells. Malic acid is found in many citrus fruits and apples. The Journal of Nutritional Medicine published a study on the combined effects of magnesium and malic acid for fibromyalgia clients. Their test used 1,200 to 2,400 mg of malic acid, with 300 to 600 mg of magnesium, for 4 to 8 weeks, with 15 clients. The results of their study showed a significant amount of pain relief within 48 hours, and a measurable decrease in pain in the tender points.[14]

Calcium and magnesium work together for proper metabolism. Calcium and magnesium must be kept in balance in a 2:1 ratio. An excess of calcium in the system will deplete magnesium levels. Magnesium is a common deficiency with those who have a high dairy intake. Milk has a calcium/magnesium ratio of approximately 10 to 1, which tends to decrease magnesium levels. Excess consumption of calcium, refined carbohydrates, alcohol, or fats can deplete magnesium. Since it is recommended to take 350 to 400 mg. of magnesium, the equivalent amount of calcium would be between 700 to 800 mg. to be in balance.

The need for **potassium** may be increased if too much magnesium is taken at once. Potassium deficiency can cause severe muscle cramps, restlessness, and irregular heart beats. Cramps can quickly be released with the use of 100-200 mg of potassium in tablet form. Fruit and vegetables juices contain 200-500 mg of potassium per cup, depending on the type of fruit or vegetables used. A whole banana contains around 390 mg. of potassium. A high amount of potassium is also found in oranges, potato peelings, and kelp. Potassium is depleted by sweating, or by using diuretic substances such as medications or caffeine.

Sodium must be kept in balance with potassium. Sodium retains fluids, while potassium is a diuretic. Organic sodium is found in many fruits and vegetables especially celery and kelp. Organic sodium is not the same as table salt, or inorganic sodium chloride. Both organic sodium and potassium are essential for proper nerve function, especially of the heart. An imbalance of organic sodium and potassium can cause nerve symptoms such as muscle discomfort, restlessness, twitching and chronic fatigue. Additionally, potassium cannot be held in the tissues without adequate magnesium. So all four minerals: calcium, magnesium, sodium and potassium must be in balance as a group, and an excess of any one of them may do as much if not more damage than a deficiency.

Trace minerals assist in the absorption of the macrominerals. For example, calcium is absorbed well when it is combined with magnesium, phosphorus, and the trace minerals manganese, iron, silicon, and zinc. Manganese helps carry oxygen throughout the body and strengthens the connective tissues. It is a mineral found in whole grains, nuts, and egg yolks. Iron is a component of red blood cells, and helps get oxygen into the blood and muscles. Iron is found in beef liver, kelp, and molasses. Silicon is a mineral that helps in strengthening nails, hair, and teeth. It is a trace mineral that is important for the brain and nervous system, and is found in green leafy vegetables, apples, almonds, and sunflower seeds. Zinc is another trace mineral that is needed by the immune system. It helps in wound healing, the formation of DNA and protein, and improves hormonal function. Zinc is found in sunflower seeds and nuts.

A few other important trace minerals are iodine, sulfur, and selenium. Iodine is needed by the thyroid to create hormones. Iodine helps prevent wrinkles, and helps in the circulation of the lymph and blood. Iodine is found in kelp. Sulfur is a trace mineral that helps dissolve built up acids. It can normalize erratic heart rhythm, and helps form amino acids and proteins. Sulfur is found in garlic, many types of berries and green leafy vegetables. Selenium is an antioxidant trace mineral. It helps prevent damage to the red blood cells. Selenium is found in onions, milk, eggs, garlic, and kelp.

Other nutrients important to help minerals be more effective are B-complex vitamins. B-complex vitamins include Thiamine (B1), Riboflavin (B2), Niacin (B3), Pantothenic Acid (B5), Pyridoxine (B6), Folic Acid (B9), and Cobalamin (B12). They are found together in nature, and support the nervous system, control anemia, help with memory, and relieve dizziness, headaches, and insomnia. B complex vitamins are found in many nuts, legumes, and protein foods, like meat and dairy foods. When using supplements, it is best to use B-vitamins in a complex, or combined form. They work better together and are absorbed more efficiently when taken together.

Obviously, minerals need other minerals and vitamins to work effectively. Notice that there are a few common foods that contain many minerals. Garlic is one of those foods. Garlic has many minerals and phytochemicals. That is why it helps improve the functioning of the immune system and is known as the poor man's antibiotic. Kelp is a type of seaweed that contains many types of minerals. Dark green kelp has many antioxidants, all of the macrominerals and many of the trace minerals. It is one of the best whole food supplements that can be used to get the full complement of minerals you need each day.

---

[14] Abraham, GE, Flechas JD, *Management of Fibromyalgia: Rationale for the Use of Magnesium and Malic Acid*, Journal of Nutritional Medicine., 1992;3:49-59.

৵17৵

Enzymes in Chemical Reactions

Enzymes are chemical substances produced in living organisms that are essential to life. They are the power needed for nearly all chemical reactions that take place in the body. Enzymes work with vitamins and minerals to activate their actions. Taking supplements without enzymes will use up some of the body's enzyme reserves. Often enzymes have been compared to the electricity in the wiring system of a home. The entire lighting system (light fixtures, wall switches and wires) can be installed, yet without electricity, nothing works. This is similar to eating carbohydrates, fats, and proteins with vitamins and minerals; yet, if there are no enzymes available, the food that is eaten is not used effectively. The reason that many people take supplements, but wonder why they do not feel better, is because their enzyme reserves have not been able to break down the supplements into usable form.

Enzymes have many actions and do specific tasks. In the liver, enzymes help digest food, clean the blood, and detoxify the body. Enzymes help to build muscle by breaking down proteins in food and help strengthen the immune system. Enzymes also help the lungs by getting rid of carbon dioxide, and then reduce stress on the joints and other organs by improving metabolism.

There are actually three types of enzymes. The two types found in the body are called digestive enzymes and metabolic enzymes. The pancreas and other digestive organs secrete digestive enzymes. Metabolic enzymes are found in the joints, blood, tissues and other organs. The third type of enzymes, found in raw fruits and vegetables, are called food enzymes.

Metabolic enzymes are found throughout the body, in the blood, liver, and kidneys. Metabolic enzymes strengthen the immune system and detoxify the body. These are the enzymes that take nutrients and create muscles, bones, nails and hair. In the blood they work with the white blood cells to break down toxins. In the liver and kidneys, metabolic enzymes help keep the body functioning efficiently. The joints need enzymes to keep the cartilage strong, and the bones and nerves need metabolic enzymes to regenerate properly.

There are thousands of metabolic enzymes, however the ones needed for digestive metabolism are the most common. Digestive enzymes are needed to help break down cooked foods and carry nutrients to the cells. Digestive enzymes are sent from the pancreas to the stomach and small intestines to digest the foods we eat. The presence of gas, bloating, or other digestive disturbances is an indication that our digestive enzymes reserves are suffering. Eating more raw foods and/or taking enzyme supplements are recommended so these digestive problems will decrease.

The first step in the digestive process is chewing your food. When chewing, a salivary enzyme called amylase is activated. It helps digest the carbohydrates we eat. Then in the stomach, there are three enzymes that assist in breaking down the food into chyme. These three enzymes in the stomach are pepsin, lipase and cathepsin. The small intestine has even more enzymes to break down the chyme into nutrients. The common enzymes in the small intestine are maltase, sucrase, lactase, dipeptidase and saccharidases. In the pancreas additional enzymes, such as trypsin, chymotrypsin, pancreatic amylase and pancreatic lipase, are secreted to help the small intestine get nutrients to the cells.

Raw fruits and vegetables contain food enzymes. However, when foods are heated above 118°F, food enzymes are destroyed, and our bodies have to use our enzyme reserves to help break down foods efficiently. Over time, with the continued stress on our enzyme reserves, our pancreas actually enlarges as it tries to do its function. To support the pancreas, our digestive system will borrow the metabolic enzymes found in the blood, organs and tissues to help break down these cooked foods.

Certain fruits and vegetables are actually easier to digest when they have been steamed lightly. Especially for vegetables that are hard to chew because they are more fibrous. For example, broccoli is more easily digested when the stalks are lightly steamed for about 10 minutes. This short cooking period breaks down some of the cellulose and helps the nutrients be more easily absorbed. When vegetables are steamed it helps to break down the starches so that they are more easily digested, especially for those who have weak digestive systems. A quick steaming process does destroy only some of the enzymes, while maintaining many of the nutrients.

The most common food enzymes are: amylase to digest carbohydrates, protease to digest proteins, lipase to digest fats, cellulase to digest fiber, and sucrase, lactase and maltase to digest sugars. When we are deficient in certain enzymes, we tend to have certain symptoms related to these deficiencies. The following is a short list of common symptoms of enzymes deficiencies:

Some common symptoms of amylase deficiency are
- moist skin rashes,
- depression,
- allergies,
- hot flashes,
- cold extremities,
- neck/shoulder pain, and
- mood swings.

Symptoms common to protease deficiency are:
- back weakness,
- constipation,
- insomnia,
- hypoglycemia,
- dry skin rashes,
- acidity, and
- hypertension.

Symptoms common to lipase deficiency are:
- aching feet,
- acne,
- diarrhea,
- gall stones, and
- diabetes.

Common symptoms of sucrase and lactase deficiency are:
- hypoglycemia,
- gluten intolerance,
- moist eczema,
- diarrhea,
- asthma, and
- anxiety.

By eating foods with enzymes we reduce the stress on our digestive process, assisting the whole body to be healthier. Yet, if we maintain the standard American diet, we often miss eating any raw foods that contain enzymes. Then the body has to compensate by stealing enzymes from the other tissues and blood. This is done to aid the digestive process, since the body depends on the digestive system to get the nutrients to stay alive.

Some scientists say that the secretion of hydrochloric acid in the stomach destroys supplemental enzymes, which are then inactivated when they get to the small intestine. However, studies at Northwestern University show that 85% of supplemental enzymes are still effective when they reach the small intestine. Many types of supplemental food enzyme formulas are available that help with general digestive imbalances.

Getting enzymes in the daily diet, either by eating raw foods or in supplementation, will help to reduce oxidative stress and support the digestive system. The noticeable benefits of taking enzymes are better bowel movements, less indigestion, no bloating or flatulence, no heartburn, and better joint flexibility. For fibromyalgia patients, enzyme supplementation will help to reduce the pain, as the digestive, immune, and nervous system all begin to work more effectively. Enzymes are needed by minerals to get the stress out of the muscles. Improvements in health will gradually occur as the body heals from the inside out and the body becomes physically stronger.

❧18❧

Essential Fatty Acids and Cell Nutrition

If you have dry skin, stiffness, concentration problems, or hormonal imbalances you may be lacking in a type of fat that is essential to health. Essential fatty acids are those fats that the body needs, yet it cannot synthesize itself. Fatty acids are the building blocks of fats. Although many types of fat are unhealthy fats, some are beneficial and necessary. In fact, cutting all fat from the diet is actually harmful to health.

Essential fatty acids are critical in the proper metabolism of fats. Yet, the standard American diet mainly consists of fats that are deficient in these essential nutrients. Saturated fats are one type of harmful fat that are found in many types of red meat and dairy foods. Partially hydrogenated oils that are most commonly found in snack foods are even more detrimental to health. These types of fats, found in most vegetable oils, are converted to trans-fatty acids when heated, or oxidized. These are the types of fat that increase cholesterol in the arteries. These trans-fatty acids are not utilized by the body, and are linked to many negative and serious health conditions, such as heart disease and cancer.

Essential fatty acids are important in many metabolic processes, including energy production. Since the body cannot produce them, they must be consumed in the diet to optimize health. The essential fatty acids are the omega-3 (linoleic) and omega-6 (linolenic) fatty acids. These nutrients are the main structural components of the body's cell membranes, are crucial to optimum performance, and can enhance overall health if they are present in adequate quantities. Omega-3 and omega-6 are also crucial in preventing damage from other fats.

Omega-3 and omega-6 are the two polyunsaturated fatty acids that are necessary to produce prostaglandins, hormone-like substances, which regulate many functions in the body. Prostaglandins consistently control every cell in the body and are required for energy production. Prostaglandins increase the metabolic rate and stamina, and decrease recovery time from fatigue. Essential fatty acids help to form the structural part of all cell membranes, regulate the flow of substances into and out of the cells, and protect the cells from invading bacteria, viruses, allergens, and other toxins. Essential fatty acids are especially needed for proper brain functioning.

Every cell in the body is like a tiny factory, taking in raw materials from the surrounding fluid and sending out various chemicals. Everything going into or coming out of the cell has to pass through the cell's membrane. The membrane depends on essential fatty acids to remain fluid and flexible. Without them, the membrane becomes stiff and unable to do its job.

Essential fatty acids are also important in oxygen transfer and red blood cell production. They shorten recovery time from fatigue since they encourage the blood to bring vital oxygen to muscle cells and they enable the cells to more easily absorb nutrients needed for recuperation.

This is a list of the benefits realized by regular use of essential fatty acids:

- Improved cholesterol levels
- Lower blood pressure
- Improved memory
- Increased circulation
- Reduced joint stiffness
- Reduced dryness of the skin
- Improved immune system function
- Less inflammation
- Balanced hormones
- Depression reduced.

As you can see, fatty acids are essential for metabolism and health. Flax oil is the richest natural source of omega-3 fats. It is commonly used in salads in place of other salad dressings. Flax oil shouldn't be used for cooking, as high heat damages the fatty acids. Other sources of omega-3 fatty acids are fish oils from salmon, tuna, cod, and mackerel.

Omega-6 fatty acids are found in many vegetable oils such as borage, flaxseed, walnut, soy, corn, sunflower, and are especially abundant in evening primrose oil. These omega-6 acids are the precursors of gamma linolenic acid (GLA). Supplements providing GLA, such as primrose oil, helps the body make prostaglandins, the substances that help to relax muscles that tend to cramp.

Both omega-3 and omega-6 fatty acids need to be supplemented in the diet. The ideal ratio of these fats for healthy people is 2 parts omega-6 to 1 part omega-3. Since more omega-6 is used in the common diet of Americans, this ratio is often out of balance by as much as 6:1. For people who have immune system weakness, heart disease, blood sugar imbalance, and fibromyalgia, there is need to increase the amount of omega-3 fats so that the prostaglandins can get into a better balance. Increasing the amount of fish oils and flax oil will help especially get the omega-3 fatty acids into the metabolism. 2000 mg. of flax oil is usually equivalent to 2 capsules or 1 tablespoon, and is the recommended minimum per day.

The omega-3 and omega-6 need catalysts to be absorbed in the body. These catalysts are vitamins B3 (niacin) and B6, vitamin C, and the minerals magnesium and zinc. When these nutrients are not sufficient then the essential fatty acids will not be absorbed well. Also when too many saturated or trans fats are part of the normal diet then supplementation of essential fatty acids is less effective.

The omega-3 fatty acids have a vasodilation effect that enhances blood flow, enabling more blood to reach the muscle cells. More blood means more oxygen is available to those muscles, which will lead to reduced recovery time and less pain.

Other positive health effects of essential fatty acids include anti-oxidant activity, cardiovascular protection, healthy skin, anti-microbial activity and tumor inhibition. Their primary role in a healthy body, however, is in energy production. When added to the diet they are alkalizing to the system. As with most nutrients, essential fatty acids are best consumed with the other essential nutrients that our body requires.

A combination of essential fatty acids, minerals enzymes, and antioxidants, are all needed to make the metabolic changes that reverse fibromyalgia symptoms. By looking at the imbalances in the bio-chemical testing results and the reoccurring symptoms, the required need for each type of supplement can be determined.

ॐ19॰

Homeopathy and Fibromyalgia

Homeopathy is a type of science that looks at specific symptoms of the fibromyalgia patient, and matches them to a homeopathic remedy that fits the symptoms. Overall, whole food nutrition and supplementation will create the long-term changes to assist in improving the metabolism. Yet, homeopathy can provide more rapid relief from the pain of fibromyalgia, reduce stress that has built up in the system, and help begin the healing process.

Homeopathic medicine officially began in the early 1800's by Samuel Hahnemann. He was a medical doctor in Hungary that began the process of matching symptoms to the effects of natural substances. Homeopathy looks at each person's individual symptoms, and finds a remedy that matches the symptoms to improve health of the whole system. Many of the principles of homeopathy are used in conventional medicine today. The "Law of Similars" is based on the principle of "like cures like". A small, diluted dose of a substance will stimulate the body to control its symptoms by healing and restoring balance. If the substances were given in large doses they would cause the same type of symptoms the person is experiencing. One example of this is using the remedy Apis for a sore throat or sunburn. The symptoms of a sore throat are burning, redness, swelling and stinging pain. The same symptoms occur with sunburn. Also the same symptoms occur with a bee sting. The remedy Apis is made from a honey bee and can be given to anyone displaying those similar symptoms. In vaccination and allergy therapy, a very small amount of the bacteria or allergen is given to stimulate the body to create antibodies to these bacteria. This is similar to the "like cures like" principle.

The following remedies most often fit the symptoms of fibromyalgia, and are chosen depending on the specific symptoms of the client. These are common remedies available in many health food stores. They come in small tubes containing tiny lactose sugar pellets that have the homeopathic remedy absorbed into the pellets. Three pellets are the recommended dosage, taken one to three times per day depending on the potency. The potencies in homeopathy are listed in X's or C's. The 6X, 12X, or 30X, and the 6C, 12C, and 30C are common potencies found in health food stores. If the number is in the lower range you will probably need to take the remedy more often to see results. With a 30X, or a 30C, potency, you may see results after just a few doses.

The most common remedy used for muscle trauma is Arnica montana. **Arnica** is an herb that can be used topically as a cream on specific areas of bruising and pain. As a homeopathic remedy, Arnica can be taken internally, in pellet form, to work more deeply on the trauma that is held in the muscles. Arnica works by improving circulation and reducing both emotional and physical trauma in the muscles. It is especially useful when an accident or other traumatic event may have caused the onset of fibromyalgia.

Another common homeopathic remedy for fibromyalgia is **Rhus toxicodendron**, which is used for stiffness that gets better once the client gets moving and when weather has an effect on the degree of pain. Rhus toxicodendron is often used to relieve pain in the joints, and works well on healing ligament strains. The Rhus toxicodendron client feels very restless and wants the stiffness and reaction to cold damp weather to improve quickly.

Bryonia is the homeopathic remedy that has symptoms opposite the Rhus toxicodendron remedy. Here, the client tries to stay as still as possible, since even the slightest motion makes the pain worse. These people tend to be very irritable and grumpy, not wanting to be touched, even though pressure on the point of pain often helps. Bryonia is indicated when there is hardness of muscle groups and headaches are common. Another indication for this remedy is when warmth makes the pain worse and cool applications feel better.

Causticum is another homeopathic remedy for soreness, weakness and stiffness in the muscles that is worse from cold and/or overuse. Pain is also worse when the weather is dry and tends to be better in rainy weather. The muscles in the legs feel contracted, tight and sore, with restlessness at night. The forearms are weak, even though they are also stiff. These clients feel better in a warm bed or warm shower.

Gelsemium is a remedy for fibromyalgia when the limbs feel heavy, dull and lethargic. Headaches occur in the back of the head and neck, and there may be dizziness. This remedy is indicated when there is a low-grade fever with much aching, similar to having the flu all of the time. Gelsemium is also designated when symptoms are worse in damp, cold, or warm and wet weather, or after exertion.

Cimicifuga is a homeopathic remedy to use when there are spasms in the large muscle groups, the body feels sore and bruised all over, and there may be jerking and twitching of the muscles. The spine feels sensitive, and there is pain especially in the back, neck and shoulders. The fibromyalgia clients that would benefit from Cimicifuga feel better with warmth and pressure, and feel worse with touch, motion, cold applications and during their menstrual cycle.

Hypericum is a homeopathic remedy that helps heal nerve pain. It is especially useful when there is numbness or tingling in the extremities, or radiating pain from one area to another. Hypericum is the Latin name of St. John's Wort, and can be beneficial when depression is an associated symptom of fibromyalgia.

There are other homeopathic remedies that may more appropriately fit different specific symptoms of the client and by referring to homeopathic books or practitioners you may get better results.[15] Homeopathic remedies are also available in formulas of two or more substances mixed together. Formulas are a more user-friendly way to use homeopathic medicines since the indications for their use are extremely clear. The use of several remedies combined in formulas provides a broad effect not available in a single remedy.

Use only one remedy, whether in a formula or as a single remedy, at a time. Single remedies are recommended when the specific symptoms are known, and when a higher potency of a remedy is desired but not available in a formula. Formula products usually contain remedies in the 3x, 6x, or 12x potencies, while people with severe pain may receive more rapid benefit from the 30c potency. Two hundred years of homeopathic clinical experience has found that the higher the potency, the more deeper and faster the medicine acts. However, the higher the potency used, the more accurate the remedy must fit the fibromyalgia client. Because of this, it is recommended to use the 30c potency when the user is very confident that the remedy picked is the correct one. The use of lower potencies, such as the 6th or 12th potency, is indicated when general symptoms are used to find the remedy, or you can consider using a homeopathic formula.

When taking homeopathic remedies, it is recommended to take as few doses as necessary. With homeopathy, taking more pellets is not recommended, but increasing the frequency of the remedy may be needed to get the full effect of low potency remedies. At first, when there is the greatest amount of pain and discomfort, the remedy may need to be taken every hour. Usually after four doses, the frequency can be reduced to every two hours. As the intensity of pain diminishes, taking a dose every four hours is common. If no improvement is noticeable after a few days, it is not recommended to take further doses of the same remedy.

Although most homeopathic remedies are in pill form for internal use, there are a select number of homeopathic remedies that are available in external applications. Some external applications are in ointments, gels, or sprays. Although they have a similar degree of effectiveness, each has certain benefits and detriments. One brand I recommend to my clients is called Traumed, made by Heel-BHI. Traumed contains a number of low potency homeopathic substances that relax muscles, ligaments, and tendons, along with remedies that improve the healing response. Some other ointments are made from a petroleum base that does not allow the skin to breath very well, but they tend to work acceptably because they are not easily washed or wiped off. Gels and sprays allow the skin to breath more, but they are more easily washed or wiped off.

Homeopathic remedies must be considered as an integral part in creating a protocol to reduce fibromyalgia symptoms. The use of these remedies will reduce stress held in the muscle tissues, and will allow the pain to be relieved in a shorter period of time. The relief of pain that homeopathic remedies can provide will make it easier to create more lifestyle changes, since you will feel better and have more energy.

---

[15] Hershoff, Asa, *Homeopathy for Musculoskeletal Healing*, North Atlantic Books, 1996, pg. 120-121.

❧20☙

Bodywork and Exercises
for Stress Reduction

Treatment of fibromyalgia requires a comprehensive approach. The doctor, client and other health practitioners together play an active role in the management of fibromyalgia. Daily nutritional choices have a great affect on reversing the chronic symptoms. Studies have also shown that light movement exercises, such as swimming, tai chi, and walking, improve muscle fitness and reduce muscle pain and tenderness. Often heat applications and massage also give relief. Patients with fibromyalgia may benefit from a combination of light exercise, massage therapy, physical therapy, and relaxation.

Massage therapy can decrease fibromyalgia pain by relaxing muscles, improving circulation, which helps to get more oxygen to the muscles and remove toxins. About 25% of the participants in the research study used massage as a method to relieve pain. Most massage sessions are from one hour to one and one-half hours long. There are basically three massage techniques that are used. Stroking is a technique done by gliding the palms and fingers over the muscles in a slow rhythmic motion. Kneading is a deeper technique where the muscles are held between the fingers and thumb and slightly lifted and squeezed in slow rhythmic movements. Friction massage uses the tips of the fingers or thumb to penetrate deep into the muscles with slow circulatory motions. These three techniques are used on different areas of the body depending on the needs and requests of the client.

Other specific bodywork techniques are myofacial release and trigger point therapy. Myofascial release works deeply in the tissues to loosen up connective, or myofascial tissue and allow the muscles to relax and improve blood flow. Trigger point therapy involves holding specific pressure points to break up lymph stagnation and reduce tender point pain.

The fibromyalgia tender points develop in basically two ways. Local injury to tissues causes tearing in the fibers of muscles, tendons, ligaments, and the tissue lining the outside of the bone called the periosteum. These tears are also called soft tissue injuries. Due to continuing stress these tears do not heal. This persistent stress in the muscles near these tender points slows the flow of blood to the injured tissue and impairs the healing response.

Many tender points correlate to the myofascial trigger points used in massage therapy. Trigger points cause pain, numbness, or tingling to radiate to another area of the body. Myofacial trigger points develop from nervous system tissues that are linked during early development of the fetus in the womb. These trigger points are used in myofacial massage to release congestion that can build up from stress or injury in the corresponding tissue areas. Normally, these points are not painful unless there is some injury to the localized area. These massage techniques are used to improve circulation in the tissues and reduce pain.

Acupuncture treatments can be very beneficial for reducing the pain of fibromyalgia without medications. Acupuncture originated thousands of years ago in China, and is based on the theory that meridians, or energy pathways, link the organs with the nervous system. By placing hair-thin needles in specific points along these meridians, the circulation is improved and the lymph is able to flow more freely. Acupuncture also stimulates our body's own painkillers, called endorphins. It also affects hormones and neurotransmitters that transmit nerve impulses so it can decrease hypersensitivity to pain.

Acupuncture is one type of energy therapy. Other techniques that work similarly to acupuncture are Shiatsu, Healing Touch and Reiki. All of these techniques are based on the flow of energy or "Chi" which means life force. Energy therapists believe that illnesses are related to blocked or irregular energy locations. By lightly touching the body in certain locations along the meridian lines our own innate healing process is stirred. These non-invasive techniques, compared to acupuncture, are effective in reducing stress and pain, and improving the healing response.

Relaxation

Finding time each day to relax the physical body and reduce mental over activity helps to relieve built up stress. Just by taking a few minutes during the day to relax in a comfortable position with no background noise can have a similar effect to getting an hour-long nap. Listening to slow meditative music can help the quiet the mind. At first, it may take some time to feel like your mind is willing to slow down, but with practice you will be able to do it more quickly.

Dr. Herbert Benson of Harvard Medical School created the relaxation response. This relaxation technique is a simple way to relax your whole body. He recommends taking 10 to 20 minutes each morning or afternoon to meditate, or when needed when experiencing acute stress. He recommends beginning with several long deep breaths. While sitting in a comfortable position, begin to focus on the muscular tension on the body, starting at the feet and gradually relax each muscle as you move up the body. While focusing on your breath and releasing tension throughout the body, feel the energy circulating throughout your body. Twenty minutes of this meditation can equal 8 hours of restful sleep.

Some clients do not realize that they are physically stressed, and how much stress is in their system. With today's technology your level of internal stress can be measured. Using a program developed by the HeartMath Institute, you can measure your physiological stress by the amount of change in your heart rate. This biofeedback software program is called "Freeze Framer." It tests your pulse from a finger probe, and as your heart rate shifts, it plots the graph of each pulse rate. The greater the change in your heart rate, the more physical stress is being held in your body. As you learn to relax and reduce your stress, the biofeedback response will change, and your heart rate variability will decrease, causing the graph to become less jagged, indicating that your whole physiology is less stressed. This program shows how quickly clients are able to bring themselves into a more relaxed state. People can practice relaxation exercises and see their stress response lowered during the exercise. This ability to become physically relaxed comes with practice, and many people will recognize health benefits from it

Exercise

Exercise is recommended for everyone to stay healthy. Exercise has many benefits for the whole body. It moves stress out of the body so that it is not held in the tissues. Exercise helps to rejuvenate the cardiovascular system by strengthening the heart, lowering the heart rate and blood pressure, improving oxygen delivery into the cells and increasing blood supply to the muscle. Exercise helps mental function by relieving anxiety and tension, increases self-esteem and improves sleep patterns. Exercise improves the muscle and joints by increasing muscle strength and flexibility, strengthening bones, and improving posture. Overall health is increased with exercise by improving immune system function, lowering cholesterol and triglycerides, enhancing digestion and elimination, and increasing endurance and energy.

Before doing sustained exercise, including walking, stretching exercises help to reduce congestion in the muscles and get the muscles prepared for movement. Warm up with a few whole body motions to get the circulation flowing before begin the stretching exercises. Stretching at the end of the workout or walk also helps to relax the muscles and move the acid out so they do not get sore.

Even though we often think we get enough movement in our lives through daily activities such as housework, our exercise program needs to include an elevation in the heart rate for a period of time. Some examples of types of exercise that are helpful, but don't make the pain worse are walking, water exercise, exercise bicycles, and Tai chi. Walking at a regular pace for 20 minutes 3 to 4 days per week can be extremely helpful to the system. Water exercise in warm water helps to relax the muscles without excess strain. Tai chi includes gentle movement exercises that increase circulation and flexibility without injury.

Simple exercise movements often help to reduce the pain of fibromyalgia. Many of the participants in the study felt better with gentle exercise. Keeping the body moving helps to reduce stiffness and congestion. Also exercise has an effect on hormones that help the body to relax and promotes better sleep. Finding a comfortable exercise program that you can stick with is essential.

❧21❧

The Importance of Water

Do you drink enough water? Seems a simple enough question, yet many people who have chronic diseases would be helped immensely by just drinking more water. Water helps eliminate the acid wastes that buildup from chronic diseases. Adequate amounts of water are necessary to maintain and improve health. In fact, it is the first and easiest change that you can make to increase energy in your cells. If you don't take in an adequate amount of water, you will be more prone to chronic disorders like obesity, constipation, nausea, headaches, asthma, arthritis, and of course, fibromyalgia. Unfortunately, not many people drink as much water as they need.

First, by not drinking enough water, you can actually cause your body to retain fluid. For many years, the most common recommendation for daily water consumption was 8 full 8-ounce glasses. Yet 64 ounces per day may not be enough for everyone. Now the recommendation is to get one-half your weight in ounces per day of water. For example if you weigh 150 pounds, you would need to drink 75 ounces of water (only counting pure water) per day. Drinking coffee in the morning, a glass of wine at lunch, another cup of coffee or a soft drink in the afternoon does not count towards the water amount. In fact, drinking coffee or a soft drink with caffeine, or an alcoholic beverage, which are all diuretics, tend to dehydrate the body. Additional water is needed to replace those types of drinks.

People who tend to have fluid retention often avoid drinking water, yet they actually should drink more water. If you eat salty or processed foods and don't drink enough water, your body will pull water from your intestines and bowel to dilute the extra sodium, causing constipation. If you drink more water, you force the stored water out of your body through the kidneys. Diuretics force stored water out of your body. The problem is that your body perceives this as a lack of necessary water and it stores whatever is still available. So unless you are drinking enough water, diuretics won't usually solve the fluid retention problem. Diuretics can also cause constipation by draining water from the colon in order to distribute it around your body because not enough water is available.

Drinking more water can eliminate excess fat. Your body uses water to transport nutrients into your blood and to take wastes out of your system. A lack of water in the tissues causes toxins and fats that are normally discharged, to remain in your body. That extra weight you think of as fat may not be fat at all. It may be fluid retention that exists to protect you from toxins that have built-up in your connective tissues. Spreading out the amount of water throughout the day is easier on your kidneys and helps to control body chemistry better in the liver. Drink only 8 to 12 ounces at a time. Drinking too much water, over 16 ounces at one time, too often, will stress the kidneys. The liver needs regular hydration to keep the oxygen level in balance in the brain.

Lemon Water

Adding fresh lemon juice to your water daily can strengthen your liver. Adding one tablespoon of freshly squeezed lemon juice to 8 ounces of water in the morning will help to activate the digestive enzymes in the liver, and regulate the amount of oxygen in the blood. Frozen or concentrated lemon juice is processed and does not contain the enzymes needed to support the liver. Fresh lemon juice contains citric acid, which is the main carrier of biochemicals in the body's energy system. Lemon juice has been known to cleanse the kidneys of small calcium stones by breaking down calcium deposits. If the kidneys are too stressed, recognized by middle back pain or frequent or burning urination, then lemon juice is not recommended. Also if the adrenals are stressed, lemon juice may not be tolerated. Yet, if the lemon juice is tolerated well, it is recommended to take it regularly three to four times during the day. This will strengthen the liver and help to balance the biochemistry of the body.

What Type of Water is Best for Me?

There are many types of water for you to choose to drink. If you choose not to drink your chlorinated tap water or your well water, there are many other types of bottled water in stores today. The amount of chlorine in most city tap water varies from day to day. To discover the level of chlorine in tap water, use a pool chemical test kit and look at the chlorine level. Very often the amount of chlorine found in tap water is so high that it is at an unacceptable swimming level, and is dangerous to drink or shower in regularly.

Chlorine is added to city water to kill bacteria and other potential organisms. But when drinking chlorinated water, the intestinal flora, the good bacteria in the colon that helps digestion of food, is destroyed. Chlorinated water destroys the essential fatty acids and vitamin E our body uses to fight free radicals, and leads to dryness in the cell membranes that lead to skin disorders and many other problems with nutrient absorption. Chlorine, when mixed with other chemicals in water, becomes a carcinogen called organochloride that alters DNA, suppresses immune function, and mutates normal cell growth.

Chlorine found in any water affects our health, from drinking it in tap water, to showering in it. Our skin absorbs chlorine into the pores when taking a shower, and in hot showers the chlorine gets into the air and is inhaled. So using chlorinated water in any form is detrimental to health, especially when there is so much chlorine in the water that a pool water chemical test kit says it is unsafe for swimming.

Well water can have bacteria in it, along with minerals and chemicals from the earth and rock from where it is drawn. The amount of minerals in well water can make the water hard, gradually building up inorganic minerals and chemicals in the fatty tissues. By softening the water with a water softener, the water makes suds better, but does not remove the bacteria, inorganic minerals, and chemicals.

Bottled water comes in a variety of forms. Some choices are spring water that really comes from a natural spring, others are carbon-filtered tap water, reverse osmosis filtered water, and steam distilled water. Bottled water has many different potential qualities. Unless you know exactly the form of the water that you are buying and have it tested for chlorine and pH, you may not know what you are drinking.

Carbon filtering takes many of the inorganic minerals, like chlorine, out of the water. It is one of the most common ways of making tap water safe to drink. Reverse osmosis water filters out most of the chemicals and bacteria, flushing the wastes out with the excess water that is discharged. This water is pure, as is steam-distilled water, which also has all the inorganic minerals removed.

Distillation is a process where tap water is boiled, evaporated and the vapor condensed into another container. For short periods of time, drinking distilled water is beneficial for cleansing, and removing toxic substances from the body. However, cleansing is not always necessary. We need to build up our mineral reserves, and by drinking distilled water consistently, we will have trouble maintaining a good mineral balance unless mineral supplements are used. One of the problems with distilled water is that it is an active absorber, and when it comes into contact with air, it absorbs carbon dioxide, making its pH reading more acid. Even though the ideal pH of water is between 6.6 and 7.4, the pH of distilled water is found to be closer to 6.0 pH. The longer one drinks distilled water, the more likely the development of mineral deficiencies and an acid state. Those who supplement their distilled water intake with trace minerals are not as deficient but still not as adequately nourished as people who drink water with minerals in it. The ideal water for the human body should be slightly alkaline and this requires the presence of minerals like calcium and magnesium.

Another choice for water is ionized water. This water separates the alkaline minerals in the tap water from the acid minerals. The common alkaline minerals found in tap water are calcium, magnesium, sodium and potassium. The acid minerals are chlorine, sulfur and phosphorus. They are the same minerals found in our foods. A water ionizer unit has two chambers with positive and negative electrodes. The negative electrode attracts positive minerals, which are alkaline minerals, to its chamber, while the positive electrode attracts negative minerals, which are acid minerals, to its chamber. The water actually undergoes a change of its electrical state.

When ionizing, the water molecule is split into two parts. The hydrogen ion (H+) is separated from the hydroxyl ion (OH-). When water has more hydrogen ions, the water tests more acid. When the water has more hydroxyl ions the water is more alkaline, or measures above 7.0 pH. Ionized water has a negative charge of -250 to -350 mV. This negative charge only lasts for 18 to 24 hours after being made and makes the water work as an antioxidant, which slows down the aging process. Minerals that are ionized are more bio-available, meaning that the body is able to absorb them more efficiently. Ionized water is an efficient and effective way for the body to get its minerals.

When choosing water to drink on a daily basis, check for hardness, chlorine content, and the pH level. Ideally pH level should be between 6.6 and 7.4 in bottled, processed, or filtered water. Any water that tests less than 6.0 is too acid to consume on a daily basis. The next section discusses the effects of drinking carbonated drinks, which can also increase acidity in the body.

~22~

What about Soft Drinks?

Soft drinks, or carbonated drinks, have become the number one consumed beverage of choice in America within the last few years. Drinking this flavored carbonated water with preservatives could be one of the most harmful habits we can have. The carbonated water alone creates carbonic acid in our system. Added phosphoric or citric acid increases the acidity of the drink. Soft drinks have a pH level between 2 and 3 pH, compared to water that has a pH between 6.6 and 7.4. Constant consumption of acid drinks increases the acidity in the body, and over the long term creates acidosis that can lead to anemia and nervous system weakness.

The carbonation in soft drinks causes acidity in our tissues. However, carbonic acid is easily breathed out of the body when the lungs are healthy. But the other additives in soft drinks cause acidity in the tissues even after the carbonation is all fizzled out. Phosphoric acid is added to many of the dark sodas to help keep the carbonation from going flat. When excess amounts of the mineral phosphorus are present in your body then calcium has to come out of the bones and into the blood to balance this phosphorus. The calcium that is lost in the body because of excess phosphorus in the system can lead to osteoporosis. When the blood circulates through the soft tissues, the excess calcium in the blood can end up in the soft muscle cells. As the cells begin to harden from the calcium buildup, the tender points associated with fibromyalgia are created. Phosphoric acid, along with citric acids found in the lighter colored soft drinks, neutralize the hydrochloric acid in the stomach that is needed to digest food. Because phosphoric acid and citric acid increase acidity, they break down tissues, creating even more acid wastes in the system.

Sweeteners, such as sugar and aspartame, are other components of soft drinks that make them more acid. One 12-ounce can contains 7 to 10 teaspoons of sugar. Excessive sugar in the diet leads to stress on the immune system, weakening of teeth, and excess depletion of vitamins and minerals received from the healthy foods that are consumed. Sugar stimulates activity in the physiology, but does not have the nutrients such as vitamins, minerals or enzymes to support this increased activity. The bacteria that naturally live in the mouth easily digest sugar. Acid is produced as the bacteria digest sugars. Cavities are formed as the results of this acid eating away at the outer layers of the teeth. Sugar can also cause fermentation in the digestive system, affecting beneficial bacterial growth and affecting the absorption of nutrients. In the digestive process excess sugar creates acid wastes. These acid wastes are either eliminated or are stored at various locations in the body. When the environment around the cells becomes too acid, the cells become oxygen deprived creating hypersensitivity to pain.

Aspartame, also known as Nutrasweet, is made from three components: the amino acid phenylalanine, aspartic acid and wood alcohol. By consuming

amounts for the nervous system hypersensitivity related to fibromyalgia pain.

Acid wastes accumulate from continued oxidative stress in the metabolic and nervous system. Acidosis appears in the body when the pH readings continue to be lower than normal, and potentially cause anemia and poor absorption of nutrients, leading to vitamin and mineral deficiencies. The chronic pain and other symptoms of fibromyalgia come on gradually, even when an initiating trauma may have set off the worsening of conditions. Therefore, the changes that are necessary to bring back health are a comprehensive approach looking at improving every system as effectively as possible.

Differential factors from the bio-chemical testing results show that indicators of predicting fibromyalgia symptoms are looking at urine and saliva pH readings, calcium, and adrenal stress numbers, specifically. The Free Radical test, indicating oxidative stress, did not show a great variance between people with fibromyalgia and those people in the control group. This illustrates that oxidative stress occurs in most people and affects the health of people differently.

The results revealed that the nervous system has a great effect on the tendency toward getting fibromyalgia symptoms. When the adrenals are stressed, and the nervous system does not respond effectively to stress, as indicated with the lemon juice in the Saliva pH Challenge test, there is a much greater tendency toward fibromyalgia. This is especially recognized when the urine pH reading is also low, affecting the overall metabolism. This indicates that fibromyalgia is a systemic imbalance caused by metabolic, nervous, and immune system disturbances.

A whole lifestyle program is most effective for relieving fibromyalgia. Adequate amounts of sleep are required so that the body can regenerate during the night. Daily stretching exercises will help to keep circulation flowing through the muscles. Learning to meditate and relax the mind will help balance stress factors. Diet of course is very important. Eating more whole natural foods will gradually improve the energy level. Eating meals that are low in fat and refined carbohydrates with moderate protein will keep prostaglandins in balance. Consume many dark green vegetables in the diet, and use supplements such as Juice Plus+, for the antioxidants and absorbable calcium they contain. Include supplements with magnesium and malic acid, along with the B-complex vitamins to reduce stress and improve circulation in the muscles. The one supplement that has made the most difference is the use of essential fatty acids in the diet. If nutrients cannot get into the cells the body will never be healthy. Essential fatty acids improve the absorption of nutrients into the cells by increasing cell flexibility and improving cell function.

Look at your specific symptoms, and see where you may have nutritional and metabolic weaknesses. Then select the supplements and dietary changes that will benefit you the most. This comprehensive program can be started in gradual steps to discover the changes as each step is taken. Or it can be implemented all at the same time if disabling symptoms need to be reversed more quickly. Fibromyalgia symptoms can definitely be reversed and managed when improvements are made to recover healthy functioning of the whole body by supporting the inherent healing ability.

Bibliography

Balch M.D., James F. and Balch, C.N.C, Phyllis A.,
Prescription for Nutritional Healing, Avery Publishing
Group, 1997.

Bland, Jeffrey PhD, *"Digestive Enzymes"*, Keats Publishing,
Inc. New Cannon. CN

Carette, S. *Fibromyalgia 20 years later: What have we really
accomplished?* J. Rheum. 1995;22(4):590-594.

Fibromyalgia Network, *Fibromyalgia Basics,*
www.fmnetnews.com/pages/basicis.html

Goldberg, Burton, *Chronic Fatigue, Fibromyalgia, and
Environmental Illness,* Future Medicine Publishing, 1998.

Goldenberg, DL, et.al. *"High Frequency of Fibromyalgia in
Patients with Chronic Fatigue Seen in Primary Care
Practice"*, Arthritis Rheum. 1990;33:381-387.

Granges, G, Zilko, P, Littlejohn, GO. *"Fibromyalgia
syndrome:Assessment of the severity of the condition 2
years after diagnosis"..* J. Rheumatol. 1994;21:523.

Gunn, Chan, M.D., *What is Pain?,* iSTOP, Vancouver, B.C.
Canada, 1999

Harris A.B., Pillay M, Moor A., *"Supplementation and
Excretion of Ascorbic Acid in Healthy Women."* Chem.
Biol. Interact. 14(3-4):371-374, Aug, 1976.

Hershoff, Asa, *Homeopathy for Musculoskeletal Healing,*
North Atlantic Books, 1996

Huges D.E. *"Titrimetric Determination of Ascorbic Acid with
2,6-dichlorophenol Indophenol in Commercial Liquid
Diets."* J. Pharm. Sci. 72(2):126-129, Feb 1983.

Lund N. et.al. *"Muscle Tissue Oxygen Pressure in Primary
Fibromyalgia"*, Scand J Rheumatology 1986;15:165-177.

Masi, AT, Yunus MB, *Concepts of Illness in Populations as Applied to Fibromyalgia Syndromes,* Am J Med, 1986;81:19-25)

Romano, TJ, et.al. *Magnesium Deficiency in Fibromyalgia Syndrome,* J Nutr. Med.1994;4:165-167.

Ronzio, R.A., *"Nutritional Support for Adrenal Function",* American Journal of Natural Medicine, 1997

Russell, J, Michalek, J, Flechas, J, et al. *Treatment of fibromyalgia syndrome with SuperMalic: A randomized, double-blind, placebo-controlled, crossover pilot study.* J. Rheum. 1995;22(5):953-957.

Santillo, Dr. Humbert, MH, ND, *"Food Enzymes",* Hohm Press, Prescott AZ, 1987

Smythe, H.A., *"Fibrositis and Other Diffuse Musuloskeletal Syndromes",* Textbook of Rheumatology 1st Edition, Philadelphia: WB Saunders, 1985, 481-489.

Resources

For up-to-date information on Fibromyalgia:
Fibromyalgia Network
P.O. Box 31750
Tucson, AZ 85751
1-800- 853-2929
www.fmnetnews.com

American Fibromyalgia Syndrome Association
6380 E. Tanque Verde Rd., Suite D
Tucson, AZ 85715
1-888-508-5524
www.afsafund.org

For up-to-date information on natural healing:
www.healthy.net
Go to their Wellness Center for articles on nutrition, homeopathy, Chinese medicine, and health topics.

HeartMath Institute
Contact for information on stress reduction techniques and the Freeze-Framer biofeedback software program.
1-800-450-9111
www.HeartMath.com

National Center for Homeopathy
801 N. Fairfax St., Suite 306
Alexandria, VA 22314
www.homeopathic.org

Chinese Medicine and Acupuncture Information
Go to traditional Chinese medicine therapy information and articles.
www.acupuncture.com

For more information on Bio-Chemical Testing:
Apex Energetics
1-800-736-4381
www.apexenergetics.com
e-mail for practitioners in your area:
        comments@apexenergetics.com

For more information on nutritional products:
Juice Plus+
Fruits and vegetables in a capsule
NSA of Memphis, TN
1-800-347-5947
www.juiceplus.com

Traumed
Homeopathic injury healing cream
Distributed by Heel-BHI
1-800-621-7644
www.heelbhi.com/bhi_traumed.html

Metagenics
Contact for very high quality nutritional supplements at
reasonable prices. Contact local health care providers.
They have Fibroplex with magnesium and malic acid,
and also a turmeric, ginger and boswellia combination.
www.metagenics.com

Sombra Pain Relieving Cream
Sombra Cosmetics, Inc.
1-800- 225-3963
www.sombrausa.com

Index